D0760351

Thieme

Direct Diagnosis in Radiology

Head and Neck Imaging

Ulrich Moedder, MD
Professor of Radiology
Director of the Institute of Diagnostic Radiology
University Hospital
Düsseldorf, Germany

Mathias Cohnen, MD
Assistant Professor of Radiology
Institute of Diagnostic Radiology
University Hospital
Düsseldorf, Germany

Kjel Andersen, MD
Institute of Diagnostic Radiology
University Hospital
Düsseldorf, Germany

Volkher Engelbrecht, MD
Professor
Head of the Department of Radiology
St.-Marien Hospital
Amberg, Germany

Benjamin Fritz, MD, DMD
Department of Radiology
University of Düsseldorf Medical Center
Düsseldorf, Germany

259 Illustrations

Thieme
Stuttgart · New York

Library of Congress
Cataloging-in-Publication Data

Kopf, Hals. English.
  Head and neck imaging / Ulrich Moedder ...
[et al.] ; [translator, Terry Telger].
    p. ; cm. – (Direct diagnosis in radiology)
  Translation of: Kopf, Hals / Ulrich Mödder ...
[et al.]. c2006.
  Includes bibliographical references and
index.
  ISBN 978-1-58890-564-2
  (TPN, the Americas : alk. paper) –
  ISBN 978-3-13-144081-5 (TPS : alk. paper)
  1. Head–Radiography   2. Neck–Radio-
graphy. I. Mödder, Ulrich, 1945- II. Title.
III. Series.
  [DNLM: 1. Head–radiography–Handbooks.
  2. Diagnosis, Differential–Handbooks.
  3. Neck–radiography–Handbooks.
  WE 39 K83h 2007a]
  RC936.K6413 2007
  617.5'107572–dc22
                              2007026165

This book is an authorized and revised translation of the German edition published and
copyrighted 2006 by Georg Thieme Verlag,
Stuttgart, Germany. Title of the German
edition: Pareto-Reihe Radiologie: Kopf/Hals.

Translator: Terry Telger, Fort Worth,
Texas, USA

© 2008 Georg Thieme Verlag KG
Rüdigerstraße 14, 70469 Stuttgart,
Germany
http://www.thieme.de
Thieme New York, 333 Seventh Avenue,
New York, NY 10001, USA
http://www.thieme.com

Cover design: Thieme Publishers
Typesetting by Ziegler + Müller,
Kirchentellinsfurt, Germany
Printed by APPL aprinta Druck,
Wemding, Germany

ISBN 978-3-13-144081-5
(TPS, Rest of World)
ISBN 978-1-58890-564-2
(TPN, The Americas)   1 2 3 4 5 6

Important note: Medicine is an ever-chang-
ing science undergoing continual development. Research and clinical experience are
continually expanding our knowledge, in particular our knowledge of proper treatment
and drug therapy. Insofar as this book men-
tions any dosage or application, readers may
rest assured that the authors, editors, and
publishers have made every effort to ensure
that such references are in accordance with
**the state of knowledge at the time of pro-
duction of the book.**

Nevertheless, this does not involve, imply, or
express any guarantee or responsibility on
the part of the publishers in respect to any
dosage instructions and forms of applications
stated in the book. **Every user is requested to
examine carefully** the manufacturers' leaf-
lets accompanying each drug and to check, if
necessary in consultation with a physician or
specialist, whether the dosage schedules
mentioned therein or the contraindications
stated by the manufacturers differ from the
statements made in the present book. Such
examination is particularly important with
drugs that are either rarely used or have been
newly released on the market. Every dosage
schedule or every form of application used is
entirely at the user's own risk and responsibility. The authors and publishers request every
user to report to the publishers any discrepan-
cies or inaccuracies noticed. If errors in this
work are found after publication, errata will
be posted at www.thieme.com on the product
description page.

Some of the product names, patents, and registered designs referred to in this book are in
fact registered trademarks or proprietary
names even though specific reference to this
fact is not always made in the text. Therefore,
the appearance of a name without designation
as proprietary is not to be construed as a rep-
resentation by the publisher that it is in the
public domain.

This book, including all parts thereof, is legally
protected by copyright. Any use, exploitation,
or commercialization outside the narrow limits set by copyright legislation, without the
publisher's consent, is illegal and liable to
prosecution. This applies in particular to pho-
tostat reproduction, copying, mimeographing,
preparation of microfilms, and electronic data
processing and storage.

Contents

9 Soft Tissues of the Neck
B. Fritz

10 Lymph Nodes
K. Andersen

Throughout the book, signal intensities in MRI and densities in CT are described in relation to adjacent tissues. In cerebral imaging, hypo- or hyperintense can obviously refer to normal white matter. However, as there are many different tissues and organs in the facial and cervical region, muscle seemed to represent the best comparison. Therefore, hypo- or hyperintense and hypo- or hyperdense usually refers to muscle tissue unless stated otherwise.

Abbreviations

ACE	Angiotensin-converting enzyme
ADC	Apparent diffusion coefficient
AJCC	American Joint Committee on Cancer
AIDS	Acquired immuno-deficiency syndrome
C1	First cervical vertebra
CEA	Carcinoembryonic antigen
CISS	Constructive interference in the steady state
CN	Cranial nerve
CRP	C-reactive protein
CSF	Cerebrospinal fluid
CT	Computed tomography, computed tomogram
CTA	CT angiography
DD	Differential diagnosis
DSA	Digital subtraction angiography
DWI	Diffusion-weighted imaging
ESR	Erythrocyte sedimentation rate
FESS	Functional endoscopic sinus surgery
FLAIR	Fluid-attenuated inversion recovery
FOV	Field of view
GE	Gradient echo
HBO	Hyperbaric oxygenation
HIV	Human immunodeficiency virus
HLA	Human leukocyte antigen
HTLV	Human T-cell leukemia virus
HU	Hounsfield unit
ICA	Internal carotid artery
I.v.	Intravenous
IU	International unit
MALT	Mucosa-associated lymphoid tissue
MEN	Multiple endocrine neoplasia
MIBI	Methoxyisobutylisonitrile
MPR	Multiplanar reformatting
MRA	MR angiography
MRI	Magnetic resonance imaging/image
NHL	Non-Hodgkin lymphoma
PD	Proton density
PET	Positron emission tomography
PRIND	Prolonged reversible ischemic neurologic deficit
SAPHO	Synovitis, acne, palmoplantar pustulosis, hyperostosis, osteitis
SPECT	Single photon emission computed tomography
SPIR	Spectral presaturation inversion recovery
STIR	Short tau inversion recovery
T3	Triiodothyronine
T4	Tetraiodothyronine (thyroxine)
Tc	Technetium
TIA	Transient ischemic attack
TSH	Thyroid-stimulating hormone
USPIO	Ultra-small particles of iron oxide
WHO	World Health Organization
YAG	Yttrium aluminum garnet (laser medium)

Definition

▶ **Epidemiology**
Prevalence of 5–10% • Common in women (up to 40%).

▶ **Etiology, pathophysiology, pathogenesis**
Thickening of the inner table of the calvarium, usually irregular, and mainly affecting the frontal bone • Benign variant • Uncertain etiology • Associated with a number of syndromes and endocrine disorders (e.g., Morgagni syndrome, Stewart–Morel syndrome) • Increased prevalence in elderly people with diabetes.

Imaging Signs

▶ **Modality of choice**
CT.

▶ **CT findings**
Irregular, sometimes nodular, thickening of the inner table of the calvarium • Bone structure is otherwise intact • No destruction or matrix changes.

▶ **MRI findings**
Calvarium thickened and hyperintense because of the fatty content of the diploë.

▶ **Pathognomonic findings**
Irregular, nodular thickening of the inner table of the calvarium.

Clinical Aspects

▶ **Typical presentation**
Almost always an incidental finding • May occur in various syndromes and endocrine disorders • Sometimes accompanied by headache due to a different cause.

▶ **Treatment options**
None.

▶ **Course and prognosis**
Benign variant.

▶ **What does the clinician want to know?**
Exclusion of other differential diagnoses.

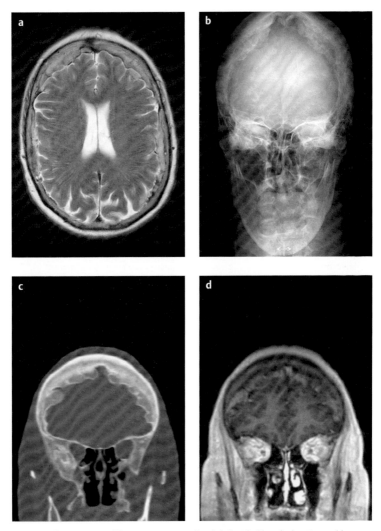

Fig. 1.1 a–d A 70-year-old woman presented with left-sided headache. General hyperostosis on axial T2-weighted images (**a**). Conventional radiography (**b**) shows irregular thickening of the calvarium. Coronal CT (**c**) and T1-weighted images (**d**) present thickened inner table of calcarium.

Differential Diagnosis

Fibrous dysplasia	– Replacement of bone by fibro-osseous tissue, chiefly in the medullary cavity, causing bone expansion
Paget disease	– Usually bilateral – Mixed osteolytic-osteoplastic new bone formation
Skeletal metastases	– For example, osteosclerotic metastases from breast or prostatic tumors – History – Scintigraphy
Hyperparathyroidism	– Hypercalcemia – Concomitant, symmetrical thickening of other bone structures
"Brush skull" appearance	– Clinical manifestations (thalassemia) – Medullary hyperplasia with radial densities in the expanded diploë and outer table

Tips and Pitfalls

Hyperostosis frontalis may be difficult to distinguish from a thin subdural hematoma based on its MRI features ● Resolve doubts by obtaining CT scans.

Selected References

Chaljub G et al. Unusually exuberant hyperostosis frontalis interna: MRI. Neuroradiology 1999; 41(1): 44–45

Dihlmann W. Computerized tomography in typical hyperostosis cranii (THC). Eur J Radiol 1981; 1(1): 2–8

She R, Szakacs J. Hyperostosis frontalis interna. Ann Clin Lab Sci 2004; 34: 206–208

Definition
....

▶ **Epidemiology**
No age predilection ● 75% of cases are diagnosed in childhood ● Cyst is usually located at the cerebellopontine angle in close proximity to the brainstem (middle cranial fossa) ● 10% of lesions are in the posterior cranial fossa.

▶ **Etiology, pathophysiology, pathogenesis**
Cystic intracranial or intraspinal mass delineated from the subarachnoid space by the arachnoid membrane.

Imaging Signs
....

▶ **Method of choice**
MRI.

▶ **CT findings**
Cerebellopontine angle mass that is isodense to CSF ● Does not enhance after contrast administration.

▶ **MRI findings**
Well-circumscribed mass in proximity to the internal auditory canal with high signal intensity on T2-weighted images and low signal intensity on T1-weighted images ● Distinguishable from epidermoid by FLAIR (low signal intensity) and DWI (diffusivity not decreased, low signal intensity, high ADC) ● Does not enhance after gadolinium administration.

▶ **Pathognomonic findings**
Mass isodense or isointense to CSF ● Complete signal suppression in FLAIR sequence ● No decrease in diffusivity on DWI.

Clinical Aspects
....

▶ **Typical presentation**
Usually detected incidentally ● May cause headache, gait disturbance, hearing impairment.

▶ **Treatment options**
Treatment is unnecessary in most cases ● Symptomatic cases are treated by surgical drainage (fenestration).

▶ **Course and prognosis**
No enlargement over time ● Treatment necessary only in cases with pronounced symptoms ● Very good prognosis ● No tendency to recur.

▶ **What does the clinician want to know?**
Diagnosis or differential diagnosis.

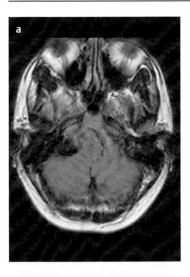

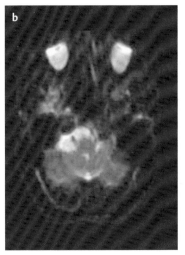

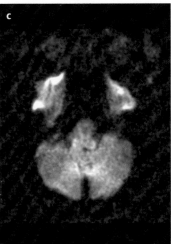

Fig. 1.2 a–c Mass isointense to CSF in the right cerebellopontine angle of a 35-year-old man. FLAIR: decreased signal intensity (**a**). T2-weighted image: high signal intensity (**b**). DWI: high diffusivity, low signal intensity (**c**).

Differential Diagnosis

Epidermoid	– Signal intensity resembles a cerebellopontine angle mass on standard MRI sequences.
	– Congenital cholesteatoma with intracranial extension
	– Nonenhancing
	– Decreased diffusivity, high signal intensity on DWI, low ADC
Cystic tumors (e.g., meningioma, schwannoma)	– Not completely isodense or isointense to CSF
	– Focal enhancement after contrast or gadolinium administration

Tips and Pitfalls

Misdiagnosing the cyst as a tumor mass.

Selected References

Dutt SN et al. Radiologic differentiation of intracranial epidermoids from arachnoid cysts. Otol Neurotol 2002; 23(1): 84–92

Kollias SS et al. Cystic malformations of the posterior fossa: differential diagnosis clarified through embryologic analysis. Radiographics 1993; 13(6): 1211–1231

Osborn AG, Preece MT. Intracranial cysts: radiologic-pathologic correlation and imaging approach. Radiology 2006; 239: 650–664

Definition

▶ **Epidemiology**
1–3 in 10 000 births ● 80% of cephaloceles are occipital, 5–10% parietal and frontal.

▶ **Etiology, pathophysiology, pathogenesis**
Extracranial protrusion of intracranial structures through a defect in the calvarium ● Meningoencephaloceles contain CSF, brain tissue, and meninges ● Meningoceles contain only meninges and CSF.
Causes:
- *Skull base and spine:* Failure of neural tube closure.
- *Calvarium:* Faulty growth induction of the bony calvarium.

Imaging Signs

▶ **Modality of choice**
MRI.
▶ **CT findings**
Bony defect with protrusion of CSF-filled meninges ● May contain brain tissue.
▶ **MRI findings**
Extension of meninges through a calvarial defect with or without brain parenchyma.
Neural tube defects:
- *Occipital encephalocele:* Myelomeningocele.
- *Parietal encephalocele:* Midline anomalies such as agenesis of the corpus callosum and holoprosencephaly.
- *Frontoethmoid encephalocele:* No associated anomalies.
▶ **Pathognomonic findings**
Prolapse of meningeal and cerebral structures through a bone defect.

Clinical Aspects

▶ **Typical presentation**
Pulsatile mass in the occipital or midfacial region ● Possible respiratory difficulties or dysphagia ● Hypertelorism ● Neurologic abnormalities in patients with associated anomalies.
▶ **Treatment options**
Surgical correction.
▶ **Course and prognosis**
Good prognosis in the absence of associated anomalies ● Otherwise, prognosis depends on the surgical outcome and other neurologic problems.
▶ **What does the clinician want to know?**
Diagnosis or differential diagnosis ● Associated anomalies.

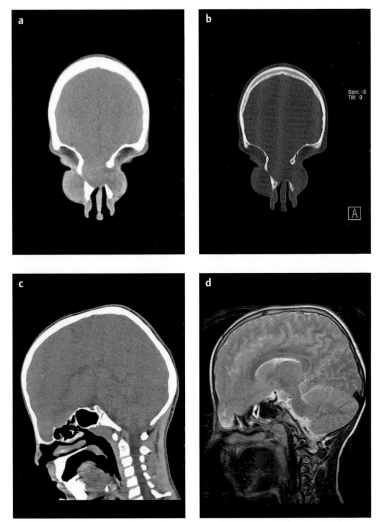

Fig. 1.3 a–d Frontobasal meningoencephalocele. The bone defect is visible on CT (**a, b**), which shows brain tissue protruding into the paranasal facial soft tissues (**c**). T2-weighted MR image (**d**) clearly differentiates between brain and meninges.

Differential Diagnosis

Epidermoid	– Fibrous connection with the subarachnoid space without a CSF fistula – Extension to the expanded foramen cecum – No extracranial brain tissue
Hemangioma, lymphangioma	– No bone defect, no extracranial brain tissue
Nasal glioma	– Tumor composed of astrocytes and neuroglia, communicates with the subarachnoid space

Tips and Pitfalls

Mistaking the cephalocele for a cystic or solid mass extrinsic to the neurocranium.

Selected References

Denoyelle F et al. Nasal dermoid sinus cysts in children. Laryngoscope 1997; 107(6): 795–800

Rahbar R et al. Nasal glioma and encephalocele: diagnosis and management. Laryngoscope 2003; 113(12): 2069–2077

Willatt JM et al. Calvarial masses of infants and children. A radiological approach. Clin Radiol 2004; 59(6): 474–486

Hedlund G. Congenital frontonasal masses: developmental anatomy, malformations, and MR imaging. Pediatr Radiology 2006; 36: 647–662

Definition

▶ **Epidemiology**
Most common before 30 years of age (75%) • 25% of cases involve the head and neck • Monostotic in approximately 75% of cases.

▶ **Etiology, pathophysiology, pathogenesis**
Replacement of bone marrow by very cellular connective tissue with irregular new bone formation • Genetically determined increase in the proliferation of poorly differentiated cells • Production of disorganized bone matrix • *McCune–Albright syndrome:* Polyostotic form with hyperpigmentation and precocious puberty.

Imaging Signs

▶ **Modality of choice**
CT.

▶ **CT findings**
Ground-glass opacity in expanded bone • Osteolytic features in cases with predominantly nonossified matrix (20%) • Sclerotic lesions (25%) • Normal appearance of the inner and outer tables.

▶ **MRI findings**
Signal intensity usually low on T1- and T2-weighted images • Possible inhomogeneous signal intensity on T1-weighted images • Inhomogeneous enhancement after gadolinium administration • Possible high signal intensity on T2-weighted images.

▶ **Pathognomonic findings**
Ground-glass opacity in expanded bone.

Clinical Aspects

▶ **Typical presentation**
May be detected incidentally • Pain • Circumscribed swelling • Craniofacial asymmetry (especially with polyostotic involvement) • Nerve compression syndrome • Spontaneous fractures (e.g., of the mandible) • Cherubism due to bilateral mandibular involvement (autosomal dominant inheritance).

▶ **Treatment options**
Surgical removal or correction is indicated only in cases with a pathologic fracture or neurologic symptoms • Radiotherapy is contraindicated, as it may promote malignant transformation!

▶ **Course and prognosis**
Spontaneous regression may occur • Lesions tend to stop growing after puberty (especially in the monostotic form).

▶ **What does the clinician want to know?**
Diagnosis • Course.

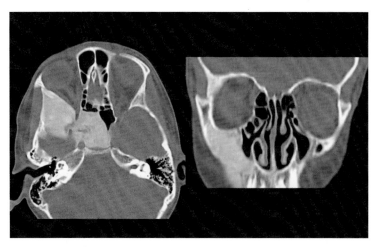

Fig. 1.4 Fibrous dysplasia of the maxilla, sphenoid, and clivus detected incidentally in a 12-year-old boy. Axial CT (left) and coronal reformation (right) show ground-glass opacity of the expanded bony structures.

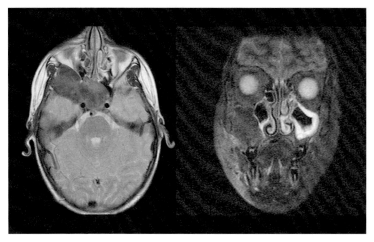

Fig. 1.5 MR image from the same patient as in Fig. 1.**4**. The thickened and sclerosed parts of the bone show a signal void in all sequences (axial T2-weighted, left, and coronal FLAIR, right).

Differential Diagnosis

Paget disease	– Involves the temporal bone and calvarium but not the facial skeleton – Inhomogeneous bone density – Combination of osteosclerosis and lytic areas
Osteomyelitis	– Clinical symptoms – History
Ossifying fibroma	– Thick bony rim – Low density of medullary cavity
Tumors (e.g., giant cell tumor, eosinophilic granuloma)	– Usually show destructive growth – May be indistinguishable from monostotic fibrous dysplasia

Tips and Pitfalls

Diagnosing a malignant tumor by MRI without taking CT scans (method of choice).

Selected References

Chong VF et al. Fibrous dysplasia involving the base of the skull. AJR Am J Roentgenol 2002; 178(3): 717–720

Kransdorf MJ et al. Fibrous dysplasia. Radiographics 1990; 10(3): 519–537

Shah ZK et al. Magnetic resonance imaging appearances of fibrous dysplasia. Br J Radiol 2005; 78: 1104–1115

Definition

▶ **Epidemiology**
Age range 5–20 years ● 60–80% of histiocytoses remain localized.
Hand–Schüller–Christian disease: Chronic disseminated form ● *Prevalence of Hand–Schüller–Christian disease in histiocytosis:* 14–40% ● *Peak age incidence:* third through fifth decades.
Abt–Letterer–Siwe disease: Acute disseminated form ● Rare ● *Peak age incidence:* first through third decades.

▶ **Etiology, pathophysiology, pathogenesis**
Hereditary, infectious, and/or immunologic etiology ● Proliferation and infiltration of lipid-laden histiocytes (Langerhans cells) in various organs and tissues ● Subsequent inflammatory response.

Imaging Signs

▶ **Modality of choice**
CT, gadolinium-enhanced MRI.

▶ **CT findings**
Circumscribed osteolytic lesion not surrounded by a sclerotic rim ● Usually has ill-defined margins ● CT shows soft-tissue component that enhances after i.v. contrast administration.

▶ **MRI findings**
Usually shows low signal intensity on T1- and T2-weighted images ● Possible high signal intensity on T2-weighted images ● Enhances after gadolinium administration.

▶ **Pathognomonic findings**
Sharply circumscribed osteolytic lesion with a soft-tissue component.

Clinical Aspects

▶ **Typical presentation**
Lesions are usually asymptomatic ● 50% are in the calvarium, 3% in the anterior skull base.
Hand–Schüller–Christian disease: Exophthalmos, diabetes insipidus, lytic calvarial lesion (10%), possible pain, swelling, fever.

▶ **Treatment options**
Curettage and cancellous bone grafting of unifocal lesions ● May respond to cortisone, cytostatic agents, or low-dose radiation.

▶ **Course and prognosis**
Eosinophilic granuloma is a benign tumor with a good prognosis (spontaneous regression) ● Curettage of spontaneous pathologic fractures ● *Abt–Letterer–Siwe disease:* Rapidly progressive course with fatal outcome.

▶ **What does the clinician want to know?**
Confirmation of diagnosis.

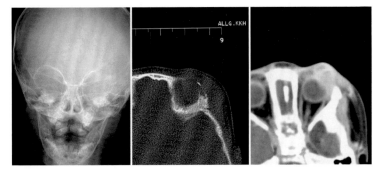

Fig. 1.6 Well-circumscribed osteolytic lesion above the left orbit with an intensely enhancing soft-tissue component (CT).

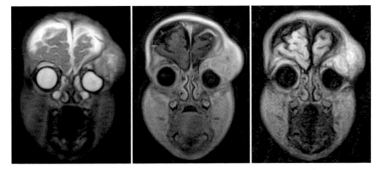

Fig. 1.7 Intermediate signal intensity (T2-weighted) with an intensely enhancing tissue component after gadolinium administration (MR image of the same patient as in Fig. 1.**6**).

Differential Diagnosis

Bone tumors *(e.g., Ewing sarcoma)*	– Permeative osteolytic area with ill-defined margins – Requires biopsy for histologic confirmation
Osteomyelitis	– History, clinical presentation – Edematous area on MRI
Dermoid	– Expansile lesion with faint marginal sclerosis

Tips and Pitfalls

Failure to consider Ewing sarcoma in the differential diagnosis.

Definition

▶ **Epidemiology**
Incidence of 2–3 per 100 000 per year ● 17% of all intracranial tumors ● 90% are supratentorial ● Peak age incidence at 40–50 years.

▶ **Etiology, pathophysiology, pathogenesis**
Benign tumor composed of meningeal cells ● Genetic causes ● Association with neurofibromatosis type 2 ● Progesterone receptor positive.
Histologic classification (WHO):
  – Approximately 90% are histologically benign.
  – 5–7% atypical.
  – 1–2% anaplastic.

Imaging Signs

▶ **Modality of choice**
Gadolinium-enhanced MRI.

▶ **CT findings**
Round or patchy mass in an extra-axial meningeal location ● 70–75% are hyperdense ● 20–25% contain calcifications ● Intense enhancement after i. v. contrast administration ● Possible bony reaction (hyperostosis) or demineralization ● Potential for extracranial tumor growth.

▶ **MRI findings**
Isointense to brain on T1-weighted images with intense enhancement after gadolinium administration ● 60% have a dural "tail" ● Variable signal intensity on T2-weighted images.

Clinical Aspects

▶ **Typical presentation**
Neurologic symptoms depend on lesion location ● Small meningiomas are often detected incidentally ● Headache ● Olfactory impairment ● Ophthalmoplegia.

▶ **Treatment options**
Surgical resection ● Stereotactic radiation may be an option, depending on location ● Preoperative embolization may be considered (to occlude blood supply from middle meningeal artery).

▶ **Course and prognosis**
Benign ● 5-year recurrence rate from 5–7% (benign meningiomas) to 75% (anaplastic meningiomas).

▶ **What does the clinician want to know?**
Diagnosis ● Extent ● Relation to neighboring structures (e.g. venous sinuses).

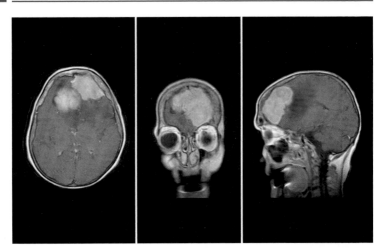

Fig. 1.8 Frontobasal meningioma shows intense enhancement after gadolinium administration. The images show a substantial intracranial mass in the skull base.

Differential Diagnosis

Schwannoma	– No dural tail
	– High T2-weighted signal intensity
Metastasis	– Bone destruction
	– No dural tail
	– High T2-weighted signal intensity
Esthesioneuroblastoma	– Location
	– Penetrates the cribriform plate and invades ethmoid cells

Tips and Pitfalls

Misdiagnosing meningioma as metastasis or malignant tumor.

Selected References

Laine FJ et al. CT and MR imaging of the central skull base. Part 2. Pathologic spectrum. Radiographics 1990; 10(5): 797–821

Macdonald AJ et al. Primary jugular foramen meningioma: imaging appearance and differentiating features. AJR Am J Roentgenol 2004; 182(2): 373–377

Turowski B et al. Interventional neuroradiology of the head and neck. Neuroimaging Clin N Am 2003; 13(3): 619–645

Definition

▶ **Epidemiology**
Constitutes 3–4% of all primary bone tumors ● Peak age incidence 50–70 years ● 35% located at the skull base.
▶ **Etiology, pathophysiology, pathogenesis**
Locally destructive midline tumor ● Originates from cell rests of primitive notochord ● Myxoid matrix around undifferentiated vacuolated cells.

Imaging Signs

▶ **Modality of choice**
Gadolinium-enhanced MRI.
▶ **CT findings**
Areas of low attenuation in bone and surrounding soft tissue ● Bone destruction (95%) ● Intratumoral calcifications (50%) and bone fragments ● Moderate enhancement after contrast administration.
▶ **MRI findings**
Low signal intensity on T1-weighted images with marked enhancement after gadolinium administration ● High T2-weighted signal intensity ● Inhomogeneities due to calcifications and intratumoral hemorrhage.
▶ **Pathognomonic findings**
Destructive, enhancing midline lesion with an extraosseous component.

Clinical Aspects

▶ **Typical presentation**
Headache ● Pain ● Diplopia ● Cranial nerve symptoms.
▶ **Treatment options**
Surgical removal combined with stereotactic radiation.
▶ **Course and prognosis**
Grows slowly ● Rarely metastasizes ● High rate of recurrence after surgical removal alone ● 5-year recurrence rate of 30–45% after proton beam therapy ● Recurrent disease has 5-year survival rate of 5%.
▶ **What does the clinician want to know?**
Diagnosis ● Extent and relation to neighboring structures (e.g., internal carotid artery and cavernous sinus).

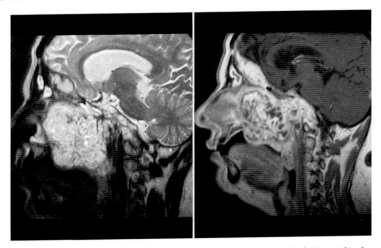

Fig. 1.9 Extensive midline tumor with typical signal characteristics: high T2-weighted signal intensity and intense, homogeneous enhancement after gadolinium administration (T1-weighted).

Differential Diagnosis

Chondrosarcoma	– Located at the petro-occipital fissure
Metastasis	– Similar imaging appearance, but midline occurrence rare
Plasmacytoma	– Possible bone destruction in the clivus
	– Low T2-weighted signal intensity

Tips and Pitfalls

Misdiagnosing as a metastasis (note relation of lesion to midline).

Selected References

Erdem E et al. Comprehensive review of intracranial chordoma. Radiographics 2003; 23(4): 995–1009

Soo MY. Chordoma: review of clinicoradiological features and factors affecting survival. Australas Radiol 2001; 45(4): 427–434

St Martin M et al. Chordomas of the skull base: manifestations and management. Curr Opin Otolaryngol Head Neck Surg 2003; 11(5): 324–327

Definition

▶ **Epidemiology**
Peak age incidence at 30–50 years • 16–33% of all paranasal sinus tumors at this age • 2% of all malignant paranasal sinus tumors.

▶ **Etiology, pathophysiology, pathogenesis**
Neuroendocrine malignancy • Arises from the olfactory nerve or olfactory epithelium (olfactory neuroblastoma).
Kadish stages:
  • Type A: Tumor in the nasal cavity.
  • Type B: Spread to the paranasal sinuses.
  • Type C: Additional spread.

Imaging Signs

▶ **Modality of choice**
Gadolinium-enhanced MRI.

▶ **CT findings**
Homogeneous mass of soft-tissue attenuation • Marked enhancement after contrast administration • Possible calcifications • Bone destruction in the anterior skull base.

▶ **MRI findings**
Intermediate signal intensity in all sequences • Homogeneous enhancement after gadolinium administration • T2 weighting clearly discriminates tumor from retained secretions • Possible cystic lesions in intracranial portion.

▶ **Pathognomonic findings**
Bell-shaped tumor extending through the cribriform plate into the ethmoid cells and the nasal cavity.

Clinical Aspects

▶ **Typical presentation**
Unilateral intranasal mass • Possible nasal airway obstruction • Epistaxis • Pain.

▶ **Treatment options**
Surgical removal • May be supplemented by radiation or chemotherapy.

▶ **Course and prognosis**
Five-year survival rate is stage dependent: 75–80% for Kadish type A, 68% for type B, 41% for type C • Resection is curative in 90% of cases • 20% recurrence rate after 8 years.

▶ **What does the clinician want to know?**
Diagnosis • Tumor extent.

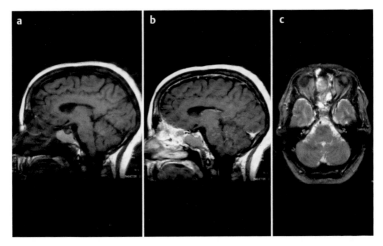

Fig. 1.10 a–c Esthesioneuroblastoma: T1-weighted image (**a**) shows a hypointense midline tumor that enhances intensely after gadolinium administration (**b**). Inhomogeneous signal intensity on T2-weighted image (**c**).

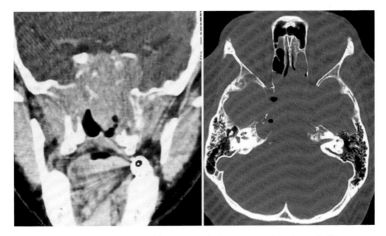

Fig. 1.11 Extensive esthesioneuroblastoma with destruction of the bony skull base. CT also shows intense enhancement after contrast administration.

Differential Diagnosis

Paranasal sinus carcinoma	– May be indistinguishable from esthesioneuro-blastoma, depending on location
Olfactory meningioma	– Dural tail
	– Rarely invades the nasal cavity or sinuses

Tips and Pitfalls

A high midline tumor of the paranasal sinuses should always raise suspicion of esthesioneuroblastoma.

Selected References

Bradley PJ et al. Diagnosis and management of esthesioneuroblastoma. Curr Opin Otolaryngol Head Neck Surg 2003; 11(2): 112–118

Loevner LA et al. Imaging of neoplasms of the paranasal sinuses. Magn Reson Imaging Clin N Am 2002; 10(3): 467–493

Pickuth D et al. Computed tomography and magnetic resonance imaging features of olfactory neuroblastoma: an analysis of 22 cases. Clin Otolaryngol 1999; 24(5): 457–461

Definition

▶ **Epidemiology**
Present in approximately one-third of the population ● Asymmetrical pneumatization occur in 5% ● Fluid retention or aeration disturbance is found in 1%.

▶ **Etiology, pathophysiology, pathogenesis**
Pneumatized petrous apex ● Congenital anatomical variant.

Imaging Signs

▶ **Modality of choice**
CT, MRI.

▶ **CT findings**
Asymmetrical pneumatization of the petrous apex (resembles the mastoid) ● Aeration disturbance, fluid retention, or fatty infiltration will opacify the cells and result in a normal appearance with an intact trabecular structure.

▶ **MRI findings**
Low signal intensity on T1- and T2-weighted images ● High T2-weighted signal intensity in cases of fluid retention ● Increasing T1-weighted signal intensity indicates increasing protein content ● DD: asymmetrical fatty infiltration.

▶ **Pathognomonic findings**
Honeycomb structure of pneumatized petrous apex ● Fatty infiltration causes high T1- and T2-weighted signal intensities on MRI with no associated mass.

Clinical Aspects

▶ **Typical presentation**
No clinical complaints ● Incidental finding.

▶ **Treatment options**
Treatment is unnecessary.

▶ **Course and prognosis**
Good.

▶ **What does the clinician want to know?**
Mass or anatomical variant.

Differential Diagnosis

Cholesterol granuloma	– Mass with high T1- and T2-weighted signal intensity
	– No enhancement after gadolinium administration
Epidermoid, mucocele	– Elliptical mass
	– Low T1-weighted signal intensity
	– No enhancement after gadolinium administration
Tumors	– Mass with low T1-weighted signal intensity
	– Moderate enhancement after gadolinium administration

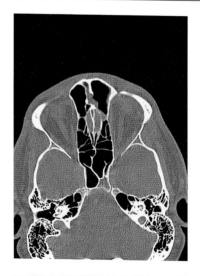

Fig. 2.1 Bilateral pneumatization of the petrous apex. CT appearance resembles the aerated trabecular structure of the normal mastoid.

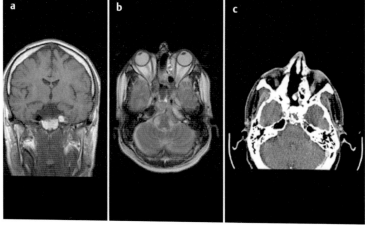

Fig. 2.2 a–c Asymmetrical fatty infiltration of the petrous apex. Detected incidentally on MRI based on the high signal intensity in the T1-weighted (**a**) and T2-weighted (**b**) images. CT (**c**) shows normal bony structure with fat-equivalent attenuation values and no mass lesion.

Tips and Pitfalls

Presumptive diagnosis of cholesterol granuloma or tumor in the absence of mass effect ● Accurate differentiation may require CT scans (intact trabecular structure!) in addition to MRI and/or follow-up.

Selected References

Greess H et al. CT und MRT des Felsenbeins. HNO 2002; 50(10): 906–919

Moore KR et al. 'Leave me alone' lesions of the petrous apex. AJNR Am J Neuroradiol 1998; 19(4): 733–738

Yetiser S et al. Abnormal petrous apex aeration. Review of 12 cases. Acta Otorhinolaryngol Belg 2002; 56: 65–71

Definition

▶ **Epidemiology**
Present in approximately 1% of the population ● Autosomal dominant mode of inheritance ● Female predominance (approximately two thirds) ● Bilateral occurrence in 80–85% of cases.

▶ **Etiology, pathophysiology, pathogenesis**
Osteodystrophy of the labyrinth ● Etiology uncertain ● Replacement of endochondral bone persisting in the petrous bone by cancellous (spongy) bone, which progressively calcifies to form plaques ("spongiosis") ● Fenestral otosclerosis is more common (approximately 85%) than the cochlear or retrofenestral form (approximately 15%) ● The cochlear form almost always coexists with fenestral sclerosis.

Imaging Signs

▶ **Modality of choice**
CT (high-resolution).

▶ **CT findings**
Circumscribed, usually punctate elliptical lucency in the petrous bone, starting at the anterior rim of the oval window ● Cochlear, circumscribed, curved, or semicircular hypodense area in the bone ● Later, progressive ossification of the oval window.

▶ **MRI findings**
May show slightly increased signal intensity on T2-weighted images ● Active disease (with bone transformation) may show punctate foci of enhancement after gadolinium administration.

▶ **Pathognomonic findings**
Circumscribed hypodensity of the petrous bone at the anterior rim of the oval window or around the cochlea.

Clinical Aspects

▶ **Typical presentation**
Conductive hearing loss (fenestral type) ● Sensorineural hearing loss (cochlear type) ● Fenestral and cochlear types may coexist ● Tinnitus.

▶ **Treatment options**
Stapedioplasty.

▶ **Course and prognosis**
Usually the progression of hearing loss cannot be halted or reversed.

▶ **What does the clinician want to know?**
Diagnosis ● DD: other possible causes of hearing loss or tinnitus.

Fig. 2.3 Otosclerosis with ill-defined spongy area near the cochlea, with increased sclerosis of the oval window.

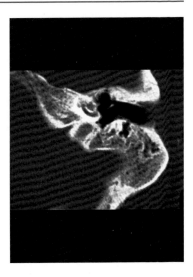

Differential Diagnosis

Fibrous dysplasia	– Homogeneous "ground-glass" density increased throughout the petrous bone
	– Increased density may spare the inner ear
Paget disease	– Diffuse involvement of the skull base in patients with mono- or polyostotic disease
	– Combination of bone destruction and repair (foci of increased and decreased density)
Postinflammatory new bone formation	– Not confined to the oval window
Otosyphilis	– Diffuse, permeative osteolytic foci

Tips and Pitfalls

Subtle lesions anterior to the oval window may be missed.

Selected References

Grampp S et al. CT und MRT erworbener Veränderungen des Innenohrs und Kleinhirnbrückenwinkels. Radiologe 2003; 43(3): 213–218

Weissman JL et al. Imaging of tinnitus: a review. Radiology 2000; 216(2): 342–349

Petrous Bone

Definition
....

▶ **Epidemiology**
Meatal atresia: 1:3300–1:10000 births ● Usually an isolated anomaly.

▶ **Etiology, pathophysiology, pathogenesis**
Congenital malformations of the external auditory canal or inner ear ● Genetically determined ● Triggered by infection or drug toxicity (e.g., thalidomide) ● Disruption of normal inner ear development (invagination of the otic pit to form the otocyst in the petrous bone; the otocyst later undergoes medial and ventral elongation and evagination to form the semicircular ducts and cochlea).

Imaging Signs
....

▶ **Modality of choice**
CT (high-resolution).

▶ **CT findings**
Meatal atresia: Area of soft-tissue or bone attenuation occluding the external auditory canal, with normal appearance of the inner ear.
Inner ear malformation: Cochlear aplasia ● Mondini malformation (incomplete cochlear development with a decreased number of turns, possible associated semicircular canal anomaly) ● Goldenhar syndrome (posterior superior semicircular canal only, expanded lymphatic duct) ● Vestibular aqueduct syndrome (enlarged endolymphatic sac) ● Michel dysplasia (complete failure of inner ear development, rare).

▶ **MRI findings**
High-resolution steady-state sequences (e.g., CISS) ● Fluid-filled inner ear structures show an anomalous configuration (e.g., cystic cochlea, absent semicircular canals) ● *Important*: Define the internal auditory canal and its structures (vestibulocochlear nerve).
Important structures to evaluate: Superior, posterior, and lateral (horizontal) semicircular canals ● Cochlea (2.5 turns) ● Normal position and shape of the ossicular chain ● Normal external auditory canal.

▶ **Pathognomonic findings**
Occlusion of the external auditory canal by soft tissue or bone ● Mondini malformation: Cystic cochlea with missing turns ● Goldenhar syndrome: Only one semicircular canal.

Clinical Aspects
....

▶ **Typical presentation**
Sensorineural hearing loss ● Secondary delay of speech development ● Microtia.

▶ **Treatment options**
Cochlear implant.

▶ **What does the clinician want to know?**
Diagnosis ● *Meatal atresia:* Normal inner ear development (ossicular chain, cochlea)? ● Normal development of neural structures?

Fig. 2.4   CT scan of the right petrous bone in a 6-year-old child shows severe inner ear dysplasia and a cystic cochlea.

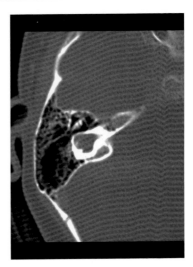

Tips and Pitfalls

High-resolution thin-slice CT scanning should not be omitted.

Selected References

Bamiou DE et al. Temporal bone computed tomography findings in bilateral sensorineural hearing loss. Arch Dis Child 2000; 82(3): 257–260

Benton C et al. Imaging of congenital anomalies of the temporal bone. Neuroimaging Clin N Am 2000; 10(1): 35–53

Graham JM et al. Congenital malformations of the ear and cochlear implantation in children: review and temporal bone report of common cavity. J Laryngol Otol Suppl 2000; 25: 1–14

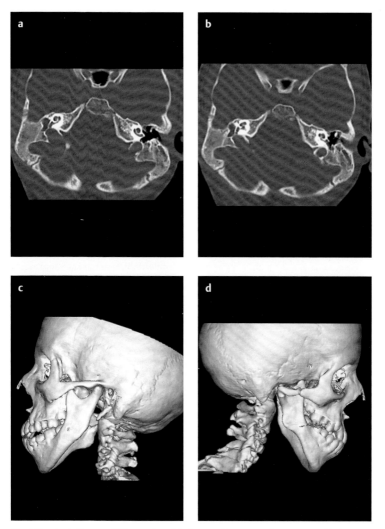

Fig. 2.5 a–d A 13-year-old boy with Goldenhar syndrome. Axial CT scans (**a, b**) show meatal atresia and absence of the auditory ossicles on the right side. Three-dimensional reconstructions of the right and left sides (**c, d**) showing absence of the external acoustic meatus on the right side.

Definition

▶ **Epidemiology**
Fractures are longitudinal in 70–80% of cases.

▶ **Etiology, pathophysiology, pathogenesis**
Usually caused by blunt head trauma ● Fractures run along lines of least resistance, often passing between fissures or foramina.

Imaging Signs

▶ **Modality of choice**
CT.

▶ **CT findings**
Scans often show an irregular linear lucency crossing anatomic structures ● Fracture lines may be indistinguishable from a cranial suture ● Extension of the fracture into adjacent structures (external auditory canal, temporomandibular joint) ● Fracture of the roof of the tympanic cavity ● Opacification of the middle ear space ● Dissection or occlusion of the internal carotid artery.

▶ **MRI findings**
Hematoma or edema of the petrous bone ● Interruption of the cranial nerves ● Altered flow signal in the internal carotid artery (MRA) ● DSA (carotid angiography) may be necessary to differentiate between dissection and occlusion.

▶ **Pathognomonic findings**
Fracture line may be longitudinal or perpendicular to the axis of the petrous pyramid.

Clinical Aspects

▶ **Typical presentation**
Longitudinal fracture: Acute hearing loss in 65% of cases (hematotympanum, tympanic membrane laceration, ossicular dislocation) ● CSF leak in 40–50% of cases ● Facial palsy, usually transient, in 20–25%.
Transverse fracture: Inner ear damage in 50% of cases (sensorineural hearing loss, vertigo, nystagmus) ● 30–50% incidence of facial palsy.

▶ **Treatment options**
Uncomplicated fractures do not require treatment ● Ossicular dislocation requires surgical correction ● Hematoma necessitates facial nerve decompression ● CSF leak requires surgical repair.

▶ **Course and prognosis**
Complications: Facial palsy ● Otitis media ● Otogenic meningitis ● Abscess formation secondary to dura mater injury.

▶ **What does the clinician want to know?**
Diagnosis ● Injury to the inner ear, cranial nerves, or internal carotid artery ● Complications.

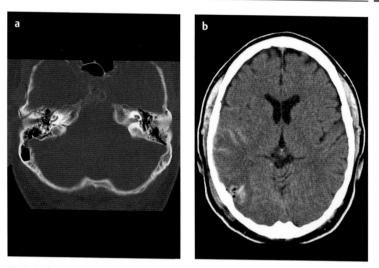

Fig. 2.6 a, b   Transverse fracture of the right petrous bone with a small hemorrhage in the middle ear. There is associated subarachnoid hemorrhage.

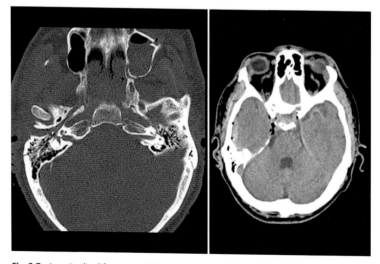

Fig. 2.7   Longitudinal fracture of the right petrous bone with bleeding into the middle ear space. The fracture extended to the posterior wall of the external auditory canal. The scans also show epidural bleeding and intracranial air.

Differential Diagnosis

Pseudofractures   – Physiological structures (compare the two sides!)
(sutures, fractures)   – Fractures terminate at suture lines

Tips and Pitfalls

Misinterpretation of cranial sutures (petro-occipital, temporo-occipital, occipito-mastoid) or fissures (tympanosquamous, tympanomastoid, petrotympanic) as fracture lines.

Selected References

Fatterpehar GM et al. Role of 3D CT in the evaluation of temporal bone. Radiographics 2006; 26 (Suppl 1): 117–132

Schuknecht B et al. Radiologic assessment of maxillofacial, mandibular, and skull base trauma. Eur Radiol 2005; 15: 560–568

Swartz JD. Temporal bone trauma. Semin Ultrasound CT MR 2001; 22(3): 219–228

Brief Definition

▶ **Etiology, pathophysiology, pathogenesis**
   - *Primary facial palsy:* Probably has a viral etiology (herpes simplex); acute peripheral damage to cranial nerve VII.
   - *Secondary facial palsy:* Secondary to neoplasia (neurinoma, schwannoma), impinging masses (especially parotid tumors), sarcoidosis, Lyme disease, cholesteatoma, or disseminated encephalomyelitis.

Imaging Signs

▶ **Modality of choice**
   Gadolinium-enhanced MRI.
▶ **CT findings**
   Scans in idiopathic facial palsy are normal • Mass in the internal auditory canal • Destruction or mass lesion of the petrous bone • Fracture passing through the facial nerve canal • Parotid tumor.
▶ **MRI findings**
   Linear or focal enhancement along the course of the facial nerve canal, especially in the mastoid portion • Mass lesion (e.g., neurinoma).
▶ **Pathognomonic findings**
   Marked enhancement after gadolinium administration in the internal auditory canal, at the external genu of the facial nerve, or in the mastoid segment of the nerve.

Clinical Aspects

▶ **Typical presentation**
   Facial nerve palsy of sudden onset • Possible prodromal signs include taste disturbance or ipsilateral facial pain.
▶ **Treatment options**
   Symptomatic treatment • Steroid or antiviral therapy • In facial palsy due to other causes, treat the underlying disease.
▶ **Course and prognosis**
   Symptoms usually resolve in days to weeks • Facial palsy persists in 10–20% of cases.
▶ **What does the clinician want to know?**
   Enhancement of the nerve • Exclusion of other causes.

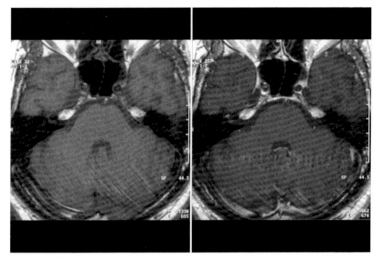

Fig. 2.8 Enhancement after gadolinium administration along the course of the facial nerve in a 15-year-old boy with acute onset of right-sided facial palsy.

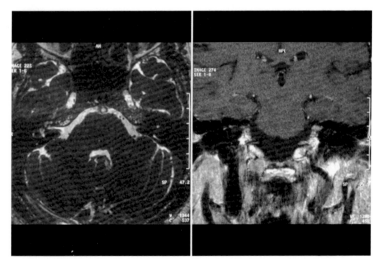

Fig. 2.9 CISS sequence shows mild edema in the facial nerve canal. Coronal image shows conspicuous enhancement of the facial nerve in its canal.

Differential Diagnosis

Neurinoma of the facial nerve	– Intensely enhancing, circumscribed mass in the internal auditory canal or nerve canal
Normal enhancement	– Slight linear increase in SI after gadolinium administration but not in the petrous bone or mastoid

Tips and Pitfalls

Failure to evaluate the entire course of the nerve ● Imaging without gadolinium ● Overinterpretation of normal enhancement ● Failure to analyze adjacent structures (e.g., parotid or skull-base tumor).

Selected References

Kinoshita T et al. Facial nerve palsy: evaluation by contrast-enhanced MR imaging. Clin Radiol 2001; 56(11): 926–932

Kress PJ et al. Der prognostische Wert der dynamischen, kontrastmittelverstärkten Region-of-interest-MRT in der Akutphase der idiopathischen Fazialisparese. Fortschr Röntgenstr 2002; 174: 426–432

Rauch RA et al. A functional imaging guide to the bony landmarks of the seventh nerve. J Comput Assist Tomogr 2002; 26(4): 657–659

Definition

- *Acute otitis media:* Middle ear infection with effusion behind the intact tympanic membrane.
- *Chronic otitis media:* Chronic suppuration of the mesotympanic mucosa • Epitympanic: Cholesteatoma (p. 39).

▶ **Epidemiology**

Acute otitis media is the second most common childhood illness.

▶ **Etiology, pathophysiology, pathogenesis**

Eustachian tube dysfunction • Causal agent in 50% of cases is *Streptococcus pneumoniae.*

Imaging Signs

▶ **Modality of choice**

CT.

▶ **CT findings**

Opacification of the middle ear space and possibly of the mastoid • Contrast administration is recommended in suspicious cases to exclude complications (cerebral venous thrombosis, associated cerebral abscess).

▶ **MRI findings**

Hyperintense fluid occupying the inner ear and mastoid.

▶ **Pathognomonic findings**

Opacification of the middle ear space with associated clinical manifestations (see below).

Clinical Aspects

▶ **Typical presentation**
- *Acute otitis media:* Pain • Fever • Hearing impairment • Onset within a few hours.
- *Chronic otitis media:* Recurrent pain • Hearing impairment.

▶ **Treatment options**
- *Acute otitis media:* Antibiotic therapy.
- *Chronic otitis media:* May require surgical treatment.

▶ **Course and prognosis**
- *Acute otitis media:* Good prognosis with complete resolution • May recur.
- *Chronic otitis media:* Recurrent effusions • Development of cholesteatoma.

▶ **What does the clinician want to know?**
- *Acute otitis media:* Complications (e.g., cavitating mastoiditis) • Gradenigo syndrome (petrous apex abscess) • Intracranial abscess • Cerebral venous thrombosis, possibly with venous infarction.
- *Chronic otitis media:* Acute exacerbation • Cholesteatoma • Intracranial complications.

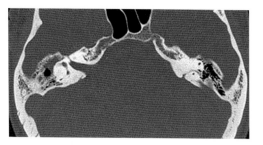

Fig. 2.10 Acute right-sided otitis media with concomitant mastoiditis in a 15-year-old girl. CT shows subtotal opacity of the middle ear space with inflammatory fluid collections in the mastoid cells.

Differential Diagnosis

Mastoid opacification due to cerebral venous thrombosis	– Thrombosis of the transverse sinus leads to obstruction of venous outflow from the mastoid – No opacification of tympanum
Malignant otitis externa	– Inflammatory process of external auditory canal (elderly diabetic patients, immunocompromised patients) – Possible bone destruction
Cholesteatoma	– Mass of soft-tissue density, usually arising in the attic region – Foci of bone destruction (erosion of lateral semicircular canal)

Tips and Pitfalls

- *Acute form:* Misinterpretation of cavitating mastoiditis • Bilateral cerebral venous thrombosis.
- *Chronic form:* Misdiagnosis of cholesteatoma • Missed labyrinthine fistula.

Selected References

Banerjee A et al. Computed tomography in suppurative ear disease: does it influence management? J Laryngol Otol 2003; 117(6): 454–458

Blomgren K et al. Clinical significance of incidental magnetic resonance image abnormalities in mastoid cavity and middle ear in children. Int J Pediatr Otorhinolaryngol 2003; 67(7): 757–760

Burian M. Entzündungen und Tumoren des Schläfenbeins. Radiologe 1997; 37(12): 964–970

Fink JN et al. Mastoid air sinus abnormalities associated with lateral venous sinus thrombosis: cause or consequence? Stroke 2002; 33(1): 290–292

Vazquez E et al. Imaging of complications of acute mastoiditis in children. Radiographics 2003; 23(2): 359–372

Definition

▶ **Epidemiology**
Ninety-eight percent of cholesteatomas are acquired ● 2% are congenital (4–20 years of age).

▶ **Etiology, pathophysiology, pathogenesis**
Cystlike mass of squamous epithelium ("ectopic skin") ● Acquired cholesteatomas develop in response to chronic otitis media ● Congenital cholesteatomas arise from ectodermal rests in the petrous bone (epidermoid).

Imaging Signs

▶ **Modality of choice**
CT, gadolinium-enhanced MRI (especially in recurrent cases).

▶ **CT findings**
Epitympanic or mesotympanic mass of soft-tissue attenuation with signs of acute or chronic otitis media.
Erosion of bony structures:
– Ossicular chain.
– Attic spur, scutum.
– Lines the tympanic cavity and invades the lateral semicircular canal.
– Infiltration or destruction of the mastoid or roof of the tympanic cavity (tegmen tympani) with intracranial extension.

▶ **MRI findings**
Hypointense mass that does not show significant enhancement after gadolinium administration ● Facial neuritis ● Acute labyrinthitis ● Labyrinthine fistula.

▶ **Pathognomonic findings**
(Epi)tympanic mass of soft-tissue attenuation with associated bone destruction (often affecting the lateral semicircular canal).

Clinical Aspects

▶ **Typical presentation**
– *Acquired cholesteatoma:* Conductive hearing loss ● Painless aural discharge.
– *Congenital cholesteatoma:* Whitish mass behind intact tympanic membrane.

▶ **Treatment options**
Surgical removal ● Mastoidectomy with reconstruction of the ossicular chain.

▶ **Course and prognosis**
– *Small cholesteatoma:* Very good prognosis after complete removal.
– *Large cholesteatoma:* Residual hearing loss ● Peripheral facial palsy ● Recurrence.

▶ **What does the clinician want to know?**
Diagnosis ● Location and extent (ossicular chain, bone erosion) ● Complications (e.g., labyrinthine fistula, intracranial extension).

Fig. 2.11 a–c

a Opacification of the left middle ear space and mastoid in chronic otitis media. CT reveals incipient bone erosion and ossicular destruction.

b, c Chronic otitis media and cholesteatoma of the right ear in a 43-year-old woman. Axial CT scan shows the middle ear space filled with chronic inflammatory tissue and erosion of the attic roof. Coronal reformatted image more clearly defines the extent of bone erosion.

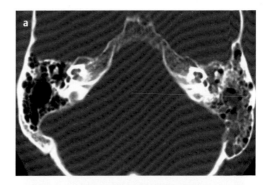

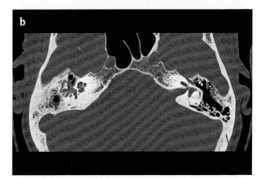

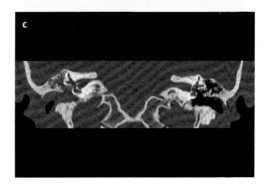

Differential Diagnosis

Chronic otitis media with ossicular destruction	– May be indistinguishable from cholesteatoma, although destruction of the attic spur and labyrinth does not occur
Cholesterol granuloma	– Mass with associated tympanic destruction – High signal intensity in all sequences due to previous hemorrhage
Glomus tympanicum tumor	– Tympanic mass that shows intense enhancement after gadolinium administration on MRI; encloses the ossicles but does not cause ossicular destruction

Tips and Pitfalls

Gadolinium administration is essential for MRI evaluation (especially in differentiating a recurrent cholesteatoma from granulation tissue).

Selected References

Aikele P et al. Diffusion-weighted MR imaging of cholesteatoma in pediatric and adult patients who have undergone middle ear surgery. AJR Am J Roentgenol 2003; 181(1): 261–265

Krestan C et al. CT und MRT des erworbenen Cholesteatoms: Prä- und postoperative Bildgebung. Radiologe 2003; 43(3): 207–212

Swartz JD et al. The temporal bone. Contemporary diagnostic dilemmas. Radiol Clin North Am 1998; 36(5): 819–853

Watts S et al. A systematic approach to interpretation of computed tomography scans prior to surgery of middle ear cholesteatoma. J Laryngol Otol 2000; 114(4): 248–253

Williams MT et al. Imaging of the postoperative middle ear. Eur Radiol 2004; 14(3): 482–495

Yates PD et al. CT scanning of middle ear cholesteatoma: what does the surgeon want to know? Br J Radiol 2002; 75(898): 847–852

Definition

▶ **Epidemiology**
Constitutes 8–10% of all intracranial tumors ● 80–90% of cerebellopontine angle tumors ● Peak age incidence at 40–50 years.

▶ **Etiology, pathophysiology, pathogenesis**
Benign, slow-growing, encapsulated neoplasm of uncertain etiology ● Arises from Schwann cells ● Most commonly involves cranial nerve VIII ● Occurs rarely in neurofibromatosis type 1 ● Bilateral acoustic schwannomas present in 96% of patients with neurofibromatosis type 2.

Imaging Signs

▶ **Modality of choice**
Gadolinium-enhanced MRI.

▶ **CT findings**
Expansion of the internal auditory canal ● Tumor enhancement after contrast administration.

▶ **MRI findings**
Intensely enhancing mass in the internal auditory canal or labyrinth ● Possible retrograde extension into the cerebellopontine angle ("ice cream cone" configuration), depending on lesion size ● Inhomogeneities or intralesional hemorrhages indicate a potential for malignant transformation.

▶ **Selected values**
– *Small tumor:* Up to 5 mm extension into the cerebellopontine angle.
– *Medium-sized tumor:* Up to 2 cm extension into the cerebellopontine angle.
– *Large tumor:* 2–4 cm extension into the cerebellopontine angle.
– Very large tumor: > 4 cm.

▶ **Pathognomonic findings**
Intensely enhancing tumor in the cerebellopontine angle or internal auditory canal.

Clinical Aspects

▶ **Typical presentation**
Tinnitus ● Vertigo ● Sensorineural hearing loss.

▶ **Treatment options**
Surgical removal ● May respond to stereotactic radiation ● If symptoms are mild, a wait-and-see approach may be taken.

▶ **Course and prognosis**
Even with large tumors, the facial nerve should be preserved ● It may be possible to preserve hearing in patients with small tumors.

▶ **What does the clinician want to know?**
Diagnosis ● Tumor extent.

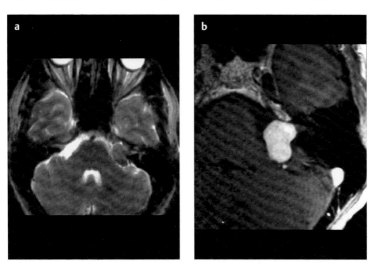

Fig. 2.12a, b MR images of acoustic neurinoma in a patient with left-sided hearing loss. T2-weighted image (**a**) shows a cerebellopontine angle tumor that is isointense to brain. The small, nodular, intrameatal tumor component is defined more clearly by T1-weighted imaging (**b**) with enhancement after gadolinium administration.

Differential Diagnosis

Meningioma of the cerebellopontine angle	– May be indistinguishable from acoustic schwannoma – Broad-based contact with the posterior border of the petrous pyramid – Does not expand the internal acoustic canal

Selected References

Bonneville F et al. Unusual lesions of the cerebellopontine angle: a segmental approach. Radiographics 2001; 21(2): 419–438

Swartz JD. Lesions of the cerebellopontine angle and internal auditory canal: diagnosis and differential diagnosis. Semin Ultrasound crMR 2004; 25: 332–352

Definition

▶ **Epidemiology**
Constitute 0.6% of all head and neck tumors ● Rarely metastasize ● Paragangliomas are multiple in 10% of cases ● 80% are glomus jugulare or carotid body tumors.
Glomus tympanicum tumors: 5:1 preponderance of females over males ● Peak occurence at 40–50 years.

▶ **Etiology, pathophysiology, pathogenesis**
Benign tumor ● Arises from chemoreceptor cells.
  – *Glomus tympanicum tumor:* Tympanic nerve (branch of glossopharyngeal nerve) ● Isolated middle ear lesion, begins on cochlear promontory.
  – *Glomus jugulare tumor:* Adventitia of the jugular bulb.

Imaging Signs

▶ **Modality of choice**
CT, gadolinium-enhanced MRI.

▶ **CT findings**
Mass in the floor of the tympanic cavity ● Only large tumors show "moth-eaten" pattern of bone destruction ● Often grows along predefined pathways (e.g., fissures) ● Only very large tumors cause ossicular destruction.

▶ **MRI findings**
Punctate foci of decreased signal intensity on T1- and T2-weighted images due to multiple vascular flow voids ("salt and pepper" pattern) ● Early, intense enhancement after gadolinium administration, immediately followed by drop-out effect (specific) ● MR venography may show infiltration of the jugular bulb.

▶ **DSA findings**
Tumor blush from large arterial feeders ● Early venous opacification ● Preoperative embolization of glomus jugulare tumors possible.

▶ **Pathognomonic findings**
"Salt and pepper" appearance on T1- and T2-weighted images ● Moth-eaten pattern of bone destruction (jugular bulb, cochlear promontory).

Clinical Aspects

▶ **Typical presentation**
Glomus tympanicum tumor: Pulsatile tinnitus (90%) ● Conductive hearing loss ● Facial palsy (5%) ● Asymptomatic vascular mass is often seen behind the tympanic membrane at otoscopy.
Glomus jugulare tumor: Mass in the neck or pharynx ● Possible involvement of the glossopharyngeal, vagus, or hypoglossal nerve.

▶ **Treatment options**
Complete surgical removal (removal of middle ear contents, mastoidectomy).

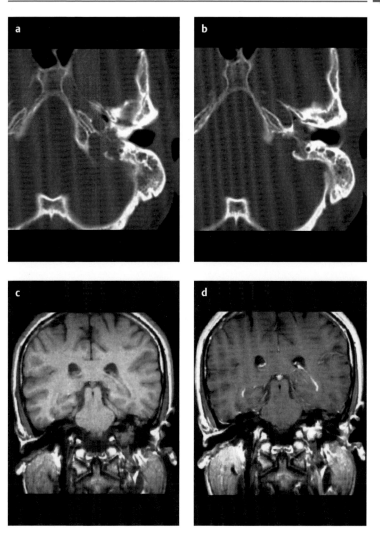

Fig. 2.13 a–d Glomus jugulare tumor on the left side. CT (**a, b**) shows a tumor mass extending from the area of the jugular foramen to the tympanic cavity. T1-weighted MR image (**c, d**) shows an isointense mass that enhances intensely after contrast administration.

▶ **Course and prognosis**
Tumor is slow-growing and noninvasive • Will not recur after complete removal • Untreated glomus tumors undergo intracranial spread, with a grave prognosis.

▶ **What does the clinician want to know?**
Diagnosis • Tumor extent.

Differential Diagnosis

High position of the jugular bulb	– No bone destruction – No "salt and pepper" pattern
Cholesteatoma	– No enhancement after contrast administration – No "salt and pepper" pattern – Ossicular destruction

Tips and Pitfalls

Variable size of the jugular foramen is not a criterion for tumor growth • Attributing a high position of the jugular bulb to a tumor mass effect • Underestimating bone erosion as a sign of glomus tumor.

Selected References

Caldemeyer KS et al. The jugular foramen: a review of anatomy, masses, and imaging characteristics. Radiographics 1997; 17(5): 1123–1139

Greess H et al. Diagnosis of glomus jugulare tumor recurrence with dynamic contrast medium flow in MRI. Fortschr Röntgenstr 2000; 172(9): 753–758

Rao AB et al. From the archives of the AFIP. Paragangliomas of the head and neck: radiologic-pathologic correlation. Armed Forces Institute of Pathology. Radiographics 1999; 19(6): 1605–1632

Van den Berg R. Imaging and management of head and neck paragangliomas. Eur Radiol 2005; 15: 1310–1318

Definition

▶ **Epidemiology**
Most common middle ear tumor in children ● Bimodal peak occurrence at 2–5 years and 15–17 years ● 50% of all rhabdomyosarcomas arise in the head or neck ● 7% arise in the petrous bone.

▶ **Etiology, pathophysiology, pathogenesis**
Very aggressive, malignant mesenchymal tumor ● *Histologic classification:* 75% embryonic, 20% alveolar (worst prognosis), 5% pleomorphic ● Possible genetic cause (mutation in *p53* gene) ● Association with neurofibromatosis type 1.

Imaging Signs

▶ **Modality of choice**
Gadolinium-enhanced MRI.

▶ **CT findings**
Inhomogeneous mass with associated bone destruction ● Irregular enhancement after contrast administration ● May contain hemorrhagic and necrotic areas.

▶ **MRI findings**
Mass of the petrous bone with high T2-weighted signal intensity ● Enhances after gadolinium administration ● Regressive changes create an inhomogeneous appearance ● Perineural tumor extension ● Intracranial extension (e.g., meningeal).

▶ **Pathognomonic findings**
Destructive mass that enhances after contrast administration ● Definitive diagnosis requires histologic confirmation.

Clinical Aspects

▶ **Typical presentation**
Often presents initially as "chronic otitis media" ● Painless (bloody) aural discharge ● Facial palsy.

▶ **Treatment options**
Surgery ● Radiation and chemotherapy.

▶ **Course and prognosis**
Grave prognosis without treatment ● Up to 80% 5-year survival rate with complete surgical removal and maximal therapy ● Potential for late recurrence.

▶ **What does the clinician want to know?**
Extent of disease (biopsy and preoperative planning).

Fig. 2.14 T2-weighted MR image confirms the ultrasound impression of a large tumor arising in the midfacial region of a 32-week fetus. A large rhabdomyosarcoma was found at postnatal surgery.

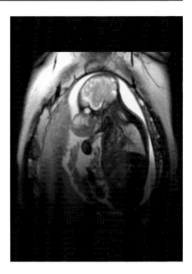

Differential Diagnosis

Cholesteatoma	– Less bone destruction – Smaller extent – No contrast enhancement
Metastases and other tumors (e.g., lymphoma)	– Age, clinical manifestations, history – Often have similar imaging features – Diagnosis based on histologic findings
Squamous cell carcinoma	– Most common malignant tumor of the petrous bone in adults

Tips and Pitfalls

Incomplete visualization of tumor extent ● Underassessment of intracranial involvement.

Selected References

Breau RL et al. Cancer of the external auditory canal and temporal bone. Curr Oncol Rep 2002; 4(1): 76–80

Durve DV et al. Paediatric rhabdomyosarcoma of the ear and temporal bone. Clin Otolaryngol 2004; 29(1): 32–37

Hawkins DS et al. Improved outcome for patients with middle ear rhabdomyosarcoma: a children's oncology group study. J Clin Oncol 2001; 19(12): 3073–3079

Imhof H et al. CT und MRT tumoröser Veränderungen des Schläfenbeins. Radiologe 2003; 43(3): 219–226

Moffat DA et al. Squamous cell carcinoma of the temporal bone. Curr Opin Otolaryngol Head Neck Surg 2003; 11(2): 107–111

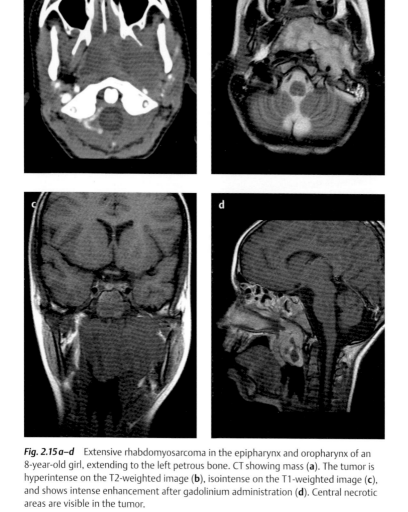

Fig. 2.15 a–d   Extensive rhabdomyosarcoma in the epipharynx and oropharynx of an 8-year-old girl, extending to the left petrous bone. CT showing mass (**a**). The tumor is hyperintense on the T2-weighted image (**b**), isointense on the T1-weighted image (**c**), and shows intense enhancement after gadolinium administration (**d**). Central necrotic areas are visible in the tumor.

Definition

▶ **Epidemiology**
Prevalence of 1:2000 ● Clinical prevalence approximately 35% in Graves disease, radiologic prevalence approximately 70% ● Peak incidence at 20–40 years of age ● Female preponderance.

▶ **Etiology, pathophysiology, pathogenesis**
Autoimmune orbital inflammation ● Associated with Graves' disease and thyroid autonomy ● Mucopolysaccharide deposition in the retrobulbar fat ● Autoimmune complexes bind to small eye muscles, inciting an inflammatory response.

Imaging Signs

▶ **Modality of choice**
MRI.

▶ **CT findings**
Findings are bilaterally symmetrical in most cases ● Exophthalmos ● Increased volume of retro-orbital fat ● Thickening of the small eye-muscle bellies may occur later in the course and is best seen on coronal reformations.

▶ **MRI findings**
Thickened muscle bellies with intermediate T1-weighted signal intensity ● High T2-weighted signal intensity in the acute stage ● Chronic cases develop low signal intensity due to fibrosis of muscle tissue ● Early involvement of the inferior rectus muscle, later involvement of the middle and superior recti.

▶ **Pathognomonic findings**
Bilaterally symmetrical thickening of the eye muscles that affects the muscle bellies and spares the tendons ● Accompanied by increased volume of the retro-orbital fat ● Relative sparing of the lateral rectus.

Clinical Aspects

▶ **Typical presentation**
Exophthalmos ● Diplopia ● Photophobia ● Chemosis.

▶ **Treatment options**
Milder cases are treated symptomatically ● Surgical decompression of the optic nerve ● The nerve can also be decompressed by irradiation ● Steroids.

▶ **Course and prognosis**
Usually runs a self-limiting course of 1 year or more ● Very rarely, leads to persistent visual impairment.

▶ **What does the clinician want to know?**
Diagnosis.

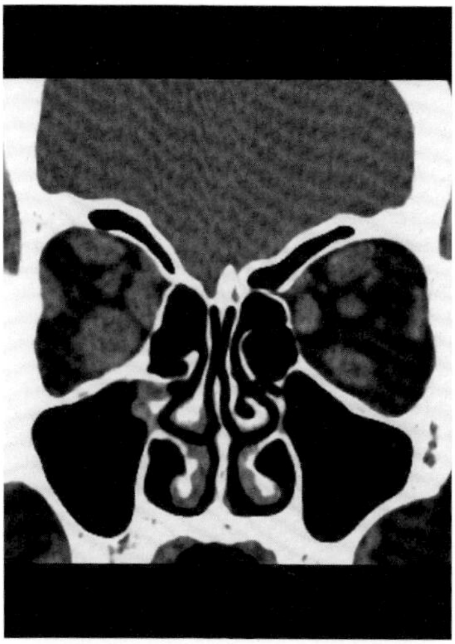

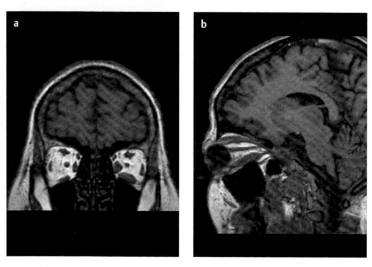

Fig. 3.1 Coronal CT scan shows bilateral thickening of the ocular muscle bellies, predominantly affecting the inferior, medial and superior recti.

Fig. 3.2 a, b Coronal and sagittal T1-weighted images in a woman with unilateral endocrine orbitopathy and thickening of the inferior and medial recti on the left side.

Differential Diagnosis

Myositis	– Not bilaterally symmetrical
	– No hyperthyroidism
Orbital pseudotumor	– Involvement of the lateral rectus
	– No hyperthyroidism
	– Frequent unilateral thickening of eye muscles
Tumor (e.g., lymphoma)	– Circumscribed mass
	– Not bilaterally symmetrical

Tips and Pitfalls

Ocular muscle thickness may not be accurately assessed on axial images.

Selected References

Cakirer S et al. Evaluation of extraocular muscles in the edematous phase of Graves ophthalmopathy on contrast-enhanced fat-suppressed magnetic resonance imaging. J Comput Assist Tomogr 2004; 28(1): 80–86

Nagy EV et al. Graves' ophthalmopathy: eye muscle involvement in patients with diplopia. Eur J Endocrinol 2000; 142(6): 591–597

Yokoyama N et al. Role of magnetic resonance imaging in the assessment of disease activity in thyroid-associated ophthalmopathy. Thyroid 2002; 12(3): 223–227

Definition

▶ **Epidemiology**

Most common in children • Peak incidence at 8 years of age • Inflammatory processes account for 60% of all primary orbital diseases.

▶ **Etiology, pathophysiology, pathogenesis**

Acute inflammatory intraorbital complication • Subperiosteal pus collection under the lamina papyracea • Secondary to sinusitis (mostly staphylococci, streptococci and *Haemophilus* species).

Chandler classification:

– Stage I: Preseptal cellulitis, inflammatory lid swelling in front of the orbital septum.
– Stage II: Periorbital edema, extraconal infiltration, periosteal reaction on the lamina papyracea.
– Stage III: Subperiosteal abscess with a normal retrobulbar space.
– Stage IV: Intraorbital abscess, intraconal cellulitis and abscess extending to the orbital apex.
– Stage V: Cavernous sinus thrombosis, direct or secondary to thrombophlebitis.

Imaging Signs

▶ **Modality of choice**

Contrast-enhanced CT.

▶ **CT findings**

Increased density of the peri- or intraorbital fat • Abscess appears as a circumscribed, hypodense, subperiosteal mass with perifocal enhancement • Air inclusions are seen in rare cases • Medial displacement of the medial rectus • Contrast filling defect in the cavernous sinus due to thrombosis.

▶ **MRI findings**

Intermediate signal intensity on T1-weighted images • Moderately increased signal intensity on T2-weighted images • Perifocal enhancement after gadolinium administration.

▶ **Pathognomonic findings**

Subperiosteal abscess • Peri- or intraorbital inflammatory component.

Clinical Aspects

▶ **Typical presentation**

Subperiosteal abscess: Swelling of eyelid • Chemosis • Pain • Diplopia • Fever. Sinus thrombosis: Severe clinical manifestations • Meningitis • Bilateral cranial nerve deficits.

▶ **Treatment options**

Specific antibiotic therapy • Surgical evacuation • Functional endoscopic sinus surgery (FESS).

Fig. 3.3 Left-sided subperiosteal abscess with marked displacement of the medial rectus and acute ethmoiditis (contrast-enhanced CT). Inflammatory thickening of the prebulbar soft tissues.

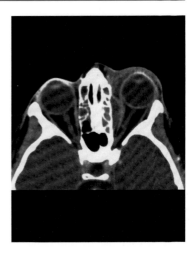

▶ **Course and prognosis**
Mortality is 17% without treatment, and blindness occurs in 20% ● Blindness occurs in 10% with delayed treatment ● 15–30% have persistent visual impairment despite adequate treatment.

▶ **What does the clinician want to know?**
Diagnosis.

Differential Diagnosis
....

Orbital pseudotumor	– No signs of inflammation
	– Thickening of eye muscles
Wegener granulomatosis	– Enhancing mass
	– No abscess
Myositis	– Unilateral thickening of individual eye muscles

Tips and Pitfalls
....

Delay in diagnosis ● Failure to obtain postcontrast images.

Selected References

Eustis HS et al. MR imaging and CT of orbital infections and complications in acute rhinosinusitis. Radiol Clin North Am 1998; 36(6): 1165–1183

Müller-Forell W et al. Entzündliche Orbitaerkrankungen. Teil 2: Bulbus, Extrakonalraum, Glandula lacrimalis, Nervus opticus. Radiologe 2003; 43(5): 400–418; quiz 419–420

Vazquez E et al. Complicated acute pediatric bacterial sinusitis: Imaging updated approach. Curr Probl Diagn Radiol 2004; 33(3): 127–145

Younis RT et al. Orbital infection as a complication of sinusitis: are diagnostic and treatment trends changing? Ear Nose Throat J 2002; 81(11): 771–775

Definition

▶ **Epidemiology**
Accounts for 5–6% of all orbital diseases ● All age groups are affected, including children ● Bilateral in approximately 30% of cases.

▶ **Etiology, pathophysiology, pathogenesis**
Idiopathic inflammatory infiltration of the orbit (synonym: idiopathic orbital inflammation) ● Nongranulomatous process affecting the orbit and its contents ● Etiology uncertain ● Diagnosed by exclusion ● Lymphocytic infiltrates ● Subdivided into acute and chronic forms, also localized and diffuse forms.

Imaging Signs

▶ **Modality of choice**
MRI.

▶ **CT findings**
Localized or diffuse infiltration of the retrobulbar fat ● Isolated or generalized, unilateral or bilateral extraocular muscle enlargement ● Enhancement after contrast administration due to hypervascular inflammatory process.

▶ **MRI findings**
Isointense on T1-weighted and T2-weighted images ● Usually enhances after gadolinium administration.
– *Localized form:* Affects only one orbital structure (eyeball, fat, muscles, or optic nerve).
– *Diffuse form:* Affects all or multiple structures.

▶ **Pathognomonic findings**
Isodense on T2-weighted images ● Diffuse infiltration of the orbit and orbital structures.

Clinical Aspects

▶ **Typical presentation**
Acute, painful exophthalmos ● Diplopia ● Visual impairment.

▶ **Treatment options**
Steroid therapy ● If unsuccessful: radiotherapy.

▶ **Course and prognosis**
Rate of spontaneous remission: 5–10% ● Good prognosis with cortisone therapy.

▶ **What does the clinician want to know?**
Diagnosis.

Differential Diagnosis

Lymphoma	– Sharp margins
	– Confined to one compartment
	– Histologic confirmation!
	– Insidious course

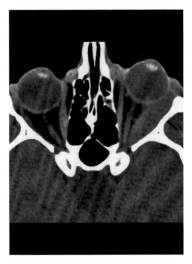 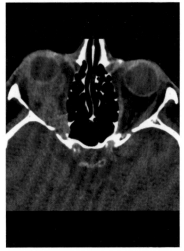

Fig. 3.4 Left-sided orbital pseudotumor with isodense thickening of the lateral rectus.

Fig. 3.5 Right-sided orbital pseudotumor with diffuse inflammatory infiltration of the retrobulbar fat.

Metastasis	– High T2-weighted signal intensity
	– Intense enhancement after contrast administration
Hemangioma, lymphangioma	– High T2-weighted signal intensity
	– Sharp margins
Myositis	– Usually affects only one eye muscle (lateral rectus)
Endocrine orbitopathy	– Early involvement of the inferior rectus muscle, later involvement of the middle and superior recti
	– Hyperthyroidism

Tips and Pitfalls

Good response to steroids does not prove lesion is a pseudotumor, because lymphomas also show good response • Histologic confirmation is often required.

Selected References

Jacobs D et al. Diagnosis and management of orbital pseudotumor. Curr Opin Ophthalmol 2002; 13(6): 347–351

Müller-Forell W et al. Entzündliche Orbitaerkrankungen. Teil 1: Intrakonalraum Radiologe 2003; 43(4): 323–334

Narla LD et al. Inflammatory pseudotumor. Radiographics 2003; 23(3): 719–729

Schlimper C et al. Radiologic features of inflammatory pseudotumors. Fortschr Röntgenstr 2005; 177: 1506–1512

Definition

▶ **Epidemiology**
Prevalence of 3:100 000 • First presenting symptom of demyelinating disease in 12–30% of cases • Approximately 50% incidence of bilateral visual impairment.

▶ **Etiology, pathophysiology, pathogenesis**
Acute inflammation of the optic nerve (CN II) • Autoimmune diseases (e.g., systemic lupus erythematosus, disseminated encephalomyelitis) • Parainfectious or viral etiology (e.g., cytomegalovirus, rubella, mumps, herpes, toxoplasmosis) • Radiation-induced (exposure of approximately 10 Gy or more).

Imaging Signs

▶ **Modality of choice**
Gadolinium-enhanced MRI.

▶ **CT findings**
CT often shows no abnormalities • Possible thickening of the optic nerve • Nerve may enhance after contrast administration.

▶ **MRI findings**
Intraorbital and intracanalicular thickening of the optic nerve • Mixed punctate and streaky enhancement after gadolinium administration (especially of the intracanalicular nerve) • Increased T2-weighted signal intensity • Sequences with combined fat and water suppression (SPIR FLAIR) are more sensitive for detecting optic nerve lesions.

▶ **Pathognomonic findings**
Thickened optic nerve showing enhancement after gadolinium administration on T1-weighted fat-suppressed imaging.

Clinical Aspects

▶ **Typical presentation**
Viral: Visual deterioration 10–14 days after underlying disease • Central scotoma • Afferent pupillary defect.

▶ **Treatment options**
Steroid therapy • Interferon is given for disseminated encephalomyelitis.

▶ **Course and prognosis**
Unilateral optic neuritis has a good prognosis with cortisone therapy • Visual impairment persists in up to 15% of cases, depending on the underlying disease • Recurrence rate approximately 20%.

▶ **What does the clinician want to know?**
Diagnosis • Intracerebral foci • Exclusion of a mass.

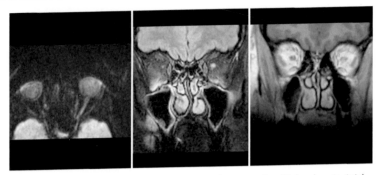

Fig. 3.6 Left-sided optic neuritis as an initial manifestation of multiple sclerosis. Axial diffusion-weighted image (left) and coronal T2-weighted MR image (center) with fat and water suppression (SPIR FLAIR) show increased signal intensity of the optic nerve. Post-contrast coronal T1-weighted image (right) shows marked enhancement.

Differential Diagnosis

Mass (e.g., optic glioma, meningioma)	– Circumscribed optic nerve expansion or mass, enhancing after contrast injection
Orbital pseudotumor	– Pain – May involve all orbital structures
Radiation neuropathy	– Rare – Prior history of radiotherapy

Tips and Pitfalls

Cerebral imaging should be done to exclude a demyelinating disease.

Selected References

Hickman SJ. Optic nerve imaging in multiple sclerosis. J Neuroimaging 2007; 17(S1): 42S–45S

Jackson A et al. Combined fat- and water-suppressed MR imaging of orbital tumors. AJNR Am J Neuroradiol 1999; 20(10): 1963–1969

Müller-Forell W et al. Entzündliche Orbitaerkrankungen. Teil 2: Bulbus, Extrakonalraum, Glandula lacrimalis, Nervus opticus. Radiologe 2003; 43(5): 400–418

Rocca MA et al. Imaging the optic nerve in multiple sclerosis. Mult Scler 2005; 11: 537–541

Definition

▶ **Epidemiology**
- *Capillary hemangioma:* Most common orbital tumor in children (1% of all newborns).
- *Cavernous hemangioma:* Most common orbital tumor in adults.

▶ **Etiology, pathophysiology, pathogenesis**
Vascular mass of the orbit:
- *Capillary hemangioma:* Benign neoplasm composed of aggregated capillaries with proliferating endothelial cells (hemangioendothelioma).
- *Cavernous hemangioma:* Non-neoplastic venous malformation with large cavities lined by endothelium.

Imaging Signs

▶ **Modality of choice**
CT, gadolinium-enhanced MRI.

▶ **CT findings**
Capillary hemangioma: Inhomogeneous mass with ill-defined margins in the upper inner quadrant • Dynamic imaging shows rapid, intense enhancement after contrast administration • Microcalcifications may be present.
Cavernous hemangioma: Well-circumscribed mass of medium attenuation • Dynamic imaging shows gradual, moderate enhancement.

▶ **MRI findings**
Capillary hemangioma: Mass in the upper inner quadrant • Low T1-weighted signal intensity, high T2-weighted signal intensity • Ill-defined margins • May infiltrate adjacent structures • Rapid, intense enhancement after gadolinium administration.
Cavernous hemangioma: Well-circumscribed mass • Intraconal in 80% of cases • Hyperintense on T2-weighted images • Isointense on T1-weighted images, enhances slowly after gadolinium administration • T2-weighted signal intensity may be decreased due to (partial) thrombosis.

▶ **Pathognomonic findings**
Cavernous hemangioma: Well-circumscribed, enhancing intraconal mass with high T2-weighted signal intensity.

Clinical Aspects

▶ **Typical presentation**
Painless exophthalmos • Diplopia.
- *Capillary hemangioma:* Upper inner quadrant • Possible extraorbital extension (bluish tumor in the eyelid).
- *Cavernous hemangioma:* Intraconal lesion with convex margins • Pseudocapsule.

Fig. 3.7 Postcontrast axial CT demonstrates an enhancing retrobulbar hemangioma.

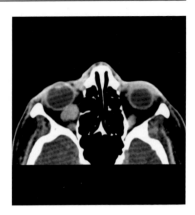

► **Treatment options**
- *Capillary hemangioma:* Observation • Steroids • Laser therapy • Surgical removal has varying results.
- *Cavernous hemangioma:* Surgical removal • High surgical risk may justify an expectant approach.

► **Course and prognosis**
- *Capillary hemangioma:* Lesion grows during the first 6 months of life • This stage is followed by spontaneous remission (50% at 5 years, 70% at 7 years).
- *Cavernous hemangioma:* Very good prognosis with complete removal.

► **What does the clinician want to know?**
Diagnosis • Extent • Course.

Differential Diagnosis

Lymphangioma	– Fluid–fluid level
	– Multifocal
Varices	– Dilated, tortuous vessel
Orbital pseudotumor	– Painful exophthalmos
Mass (e.g., metastasis, lymphoma)	– History
	– Invasive, potentially bone-destructive lesion
Rhabdomyosarcoma	– Invasive, bone-destructive lesion

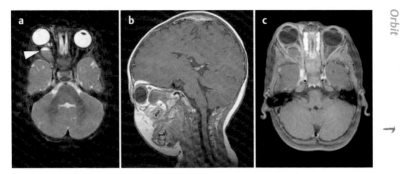

Fig. 3.8a–c Hemangioma in the right orbit, with intralesional hemorrhage (arrow: fluid level). Appearance of the extraconal mass on T1-weighted image (**a**) and T2-weighted image (**b**). Lesion shows slight enhancement after gadolinium administration on T1-weighted image (**c**).

Selected References

Ansari SA et al. Orbital cavernous hemangioma: role of imaging. Neuroimaging. Clin N Am 2005; 15: 137–158

Bilaniuk LT. Orbital vascular lesions. Role of imaging. Radiol Clin North Am 1999; 37(1): 169–183

Mueller-Forell W et al. Orbital pathology. Eur J Radiol 2004; 49: 105–142

Definition

▸ **Epidemiology**
Three percent of all orbital tumors (four times more common than meningioma) ● 66% of all optic nerve tumors ● Bilateral involvement is common in neurofibromatosis type 1 ● 10–40% of patients with optic gliomas have neurofibromatosis type 1, and 15–40% of patients with neurofibromatosis type 1 have optic gliomas ● 50–85% of optic gliomas extend to the optic chiasm or hypothalamus.

▸ **Etiology, pathophysiology, pathogenesis**
Benign neuroglial tumor of the optic nerve ● Grade I astrocytoma of CN II (glial hyperplasia).

Imaging Signs

▸ **Modality of choice**
Gadolinium-enhanced MRI.

▸ **CT findings**
Thickening of the optic nerve ● Intracanalicular involvement ● Expansion of the optic nerve canal.

▸ **MRI findings**
Iso- to hypointense on T1-weighted images ● Usually hyperintense on T2-weighted images ● Homogeneous enhancement after gadolinium administration ● The nerve is not delineated within the tumor ● All optic gliomas in neurofibromatosis type 1 involve the chiasm only, display cystic changes, and show marked enhancement after gadolinium administration.

▸ **Selected normal values**
Intraorbital length of optic nerve = 25 mm ● Intracanalicular length = 5 mm ● Intracranial length = 10 mm ● Normal diameter = 4–6 mm.

▸ **Pathognomonic findings**
Sausage-shaped thickening and kinking of the optic nerve.

Clinical Aspects

▸ **Typical presentation**
Painless exophthalmos ● Visual deterioration ● Possible nystagmus.

▸ **Treatment options**
Wait-and-see with onset at 4–6 years of age ● Radiotherapy or chemotherapy is indicated in patients with visual impairment.

▸ **Course and prognosis**
Stable course with onset after 6 years of age ● Spontaneous remission may occur.

▸ **What does the clinician want to know?**
Diagnosis ● Course.

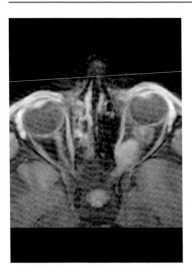

Fig. 3.9 Postcontrast axial T1-weighted image with fat suppression shows an elliptical, enhancing glioma in the course of the left optic nerve.

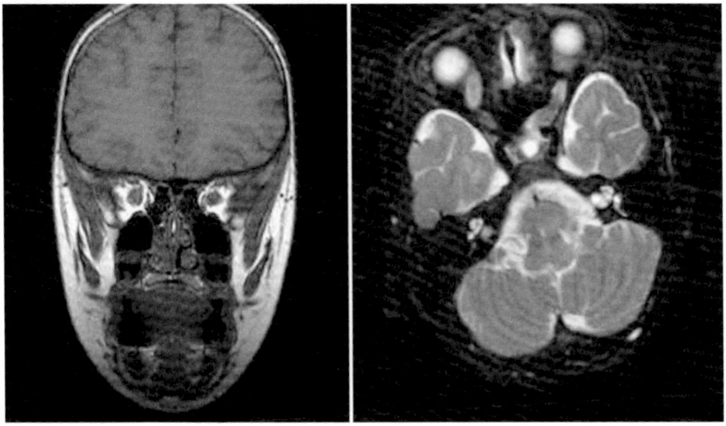

Fig. 3.10 Bilateral optic gliomas in a patient with known neurofibromatosis type 1 (T1-weighted coronal, T2-weighted axial).

Differential Diagnosis

Optic neuritis	– Nerve enhances inhomogeneously, may be thickened – association to demyelinating disease
Optic meningioma	– Nerve can be identified in the enhancing tumor – Calcifications

Tips and Pitfalls

A common error is missing tumor extension into the optic chiasm (the neurocranium should be evaluated by MRI).

Selected References

Chateil JF et al. MRI and clinical differences between optic pathway tumours in children with and without neurofibromatosis. Br J Radiol 2001; 74(877): 24–31

Hollander MD et al. Optic Gliomas. Radiol Clin North Am 1999; 37(1): 59–71

Miller NR. Primary tumors of the optic nerve and its sheath. Eye 2004; 18: 1026–1037

Schröder S et al. Long-term outcome of gliomas of the visual pathway in type 1 neurofibromatosis. Klin Monatsbl Augenheilkd 1999; 215(6): 349–354

Definition

▶ **Epidemiology**
Prevalence of 1:20 000 ● More than 90% occur in children under 5 years of age ●
70% are unilateral, 30% bilateral ● Trilateral: bilateral plus pineal or suprasellar
lesion (1%) ● Tetralateral: bilateral plus pineal and suprasellar lesions (< 0.1%).

▶ **Etiology, pathophysiology, pathogenesis**
High-grade primary malignant tumor of neuroectodermal cell origin in the retina ● Inactivation of both alleles of the *Rb1* gene on chromosome 13q14 ● Retino-
blastomas are classified as sporadic (100% unilateral) or hereditary (85% bilateral).

Imaging Signs

▶ **Modality of choice**
Gadolinium-enhanced MRI.

▶ **CT findings**
Mass within the eye ● Calcifications present in 90%.

▶ **MRI findings**
Mass within the eye ● Slightly increased T1-weighted signal intensity ● Low T2-
weighted signal intensity ● Moderate to intense enhancement after gadolinium
administration.

▶ **Pathognomonic findings**
Calcified intraocular mass.

Clinical Aspects

▶ **Typical presentation**
Leukokoria ● Strabismus ● Glaucoma ● Visual impairment.

▶ **Treatment options**
Surgical removal ● Radiotherapy.

▶ **Course and prognosis**
Small, posteriorly situated tumors have a good prognosis ● Tumors located anterior to the equator, involving more than half the retina, or with vitreous metastases have a poor prognosis.
Hereditary retinoblastoma: Association with other malignancies, especially os-
teosarcoma ● Secondary tumors after radiotherapy: 20% at 10 years, 50% at 20
years, 90% at 30 years.

▶ **What does the clinician want to know?**
Diagnosis ● Extent ● Intracerebral findings.

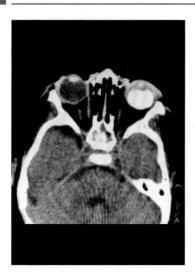

Fig. 3.11 CT scan through the orbit of an infant with a left-sided retinoblastoma. The calcified mass completely occupies the posterior portion of the eye.

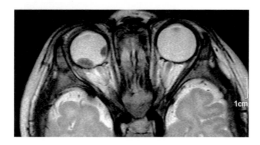

Fig. 3.12 MRI of a multifocal retinoblastoma of the right eye (low T2-weighted signal intensity).

Differential Diagnosis

Persistent hyperplastic vitreous	– Microphthalmos
	– Retrolental fibrovascular membrane with positive enhancement after gadolinium administration
	– No calcification
Retinal detachment	– Subretinal hemorrhage without calcification
	– Retinoblastoma is a possible cause!
Coats disease	– Subretinal fat accumulation
	– CT: Hyperdense subretinal mass
	– MRI: Mass with high T1-weighted and T2-weighted signal intensity
	– Nonenhancing
	– No calcifications

Selected References

Kaufman LM et al. Retinoblastoma and simulating lesions. Role of CT, MR imaging and use of Gd-DTPA contrast enhancement. Radiol Clin North Am 1998; 36(6): 1101–1117

Schueler AO et al. High resolution magnetic resonance imaging of retinoblastoma. Br J Ophthalmol 2003; 87(3): 330–335

Shields CL et al. Diagnosis and management of retinoblastoma. Cancer Control 2004; 11(5): 317–327

Definition

▶ **Epidemiology**
Prevalence of 7 in 1 million ● Accounts for 70% of all intraocular tumors ● Peak incidence at 50–70 years of age.

▶ **Etiology, pathophysiology, pathogenesis**
Malignant melanoma of the retina ● Retina is of meso- and neuroectodermal origin ● Most tumors are choroidal ● Retinal nevi are a predisposing lesion.

Imaging Signs

▶ **Modality of choice**
Gadolinium-enhanced MRI.

▶ **CT findings**
Well-circumscribed, hyperdense mass (2–3 mm or larger in size).

▶ **MRI findings**
Signal intensity depends on melanin content ● Low T2-weighted signal intensity, high T1-weighted signal intensity ● Rounded, fungiform intraocular mass ● Intralesional hemorrhage causes inhomogeneous signal intensity ● Lesion shows moderate enhancement after gadolinium administration (especially in fat-suppressed T1-weighted sequence).

▶ **Pathognomonic findings**
Intraocular mass with smooth margins ● Low T2-weighted signal intensity, high T1-weighted signal intensity ● Tumor arises from the ciliary body or retina.

Clinical Aspects

▶ **Typical presentation**
Visual impairment ● Ophthalmoscopic mass ● Pain due to secondary glaucoma ● Retinal detachment.

▶ **Treatment options**
If tumor does not enlarge, wait and see ● Surgical removal ● Radiotherapy.

▶ **Course and prognosis**
Small tumors (< 10 mm in diameter, < 3 mm thick) have a better prognosis (5-year survival rate of 85–90%) ● Distant metastases (usually hepatic) may occur even in the absence of tumor enlargement.

▶ **What does the clinician want to know?**
Diagnosis ● Extent ● Infiltration.

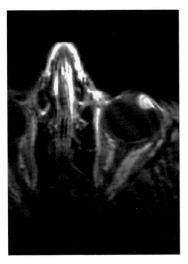

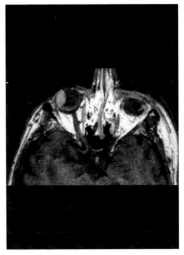

Fig. 3.13 Small melanoma arising from the left ciliary body. T1-weighted image after contrast administration.

Fig. 3.14 Advanced melanoma of the right ciliary body. T1-weighted image after contrast administration.

Differential Diagnosis

Retinal detachment	– Increased density (CT) or increased T1-weighted signal intensity (MRI)
	– Usually symmetrical, with attachment to the optic nerve
	– Nonenhancing
Senile macular degeneration	– CT: Marked enhancement after contrast administration
	– MRI: May be mistaken for melanoma
	– Histologic confirmation is required
Retinoblastoma	– Age
	– Calcifications

Selected References

Lemke AJ et al. Uveal melanoma: correlation of histopathologic and radiologic findings by using thin-section MR imaging with a surface coil. Radiology 1999; 210(3): 775–783

Mafee MF. Uveal melanoma, choroidal hemangioma, and simulating lesions. Role of MR imaging. Radiol Clin North Am 1998; 36(6): 1083–1099

Recsan Z et al. MRI for the evaluation of scleral invasion and extrascleral extension of uveal melanomas. Clin Radiol 2002; 57(5): 371–376

Definition

▶ **Epidemiology**
Five to seven percent of primary orbital tumors • Male-to-female ratio: 1:4 • Peak occurrence at 40–50 years of age • 90% result from intraorbital extension of intracranial meningioma.

▶ **Etiology, pathophysiology, pathogenesis**
Benign tumor of the optic nerve sheath • Arises from arachnoid cells • Possible association with neurofibromatosis type 1 (particularly in women).

Imaging Signs

▶ **Modality of choice**
Gadolinium-enhanced MRI.

▶ **CT findings**
Isodense to the optic nerve • Linear calcifications • Cystlike expansion of the subarachnoid space just before optic nerve entry into the eye • Homogeneous enhancement after contrast administration.

▶ **MRI findings**
Isointense on T1-weighted images • Intense enhancement after gadolinium administration (especially in fat-suppressed sequences) • Low, inhomogeneous T2-weighted signal intensity • Nerve appears hypointense in the enhancing tumor • Intracranial extension (nodular or en-plaque) • Intraorbital meningioma separate from the optic nerve is rare • Perioptic "cysts" visible on T2-weighted images.

▶ **Pathognomonic findings**
Mass distributed along the optic nerve • Enhancement after gadolinium administration • Linear calcifications (CT).

Clinical Aspects

▶ **Typical presentation**
Unilateral visual impairment • Scotoma • Exophthalmos.

▶ **Treatment options**
Surgical removal • Radiotherapy • Combination of both modalities.

▶ **Course and prognosis**
Slow growth rate • No mortality • Approximately 50% of spontaneous cases have visual loss • Postoperative visual loss is common with tumors adherent to the optic nerve.

▶ **What does the clinician want to know?**
Diagnosis • Intracranial extension.

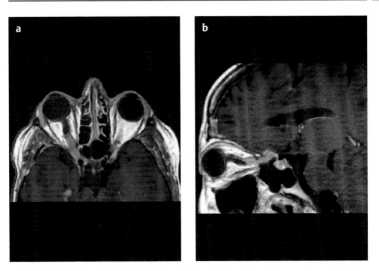

Fig. 3.15 a, b   Right-sided optic nerve meningioma. T1-weighted image after gadolinium administration shows an intensely enhancing tumor extending from the midportion of the intraorbital optic nerve to the optic chiasm.

Differential Diagnosis

Orbital pseudotumor	– Pain – Not confined to the optic nerve
Optic neuritis	– Possible thickening of the nerve – Inhomogeneous enhancement of nerve itself – Association with demyelinating disease
Optic glioma	– No calcifications – Optic nerve is not delineated
Sarcoidosis	– Thickened nerve with enhancement after gadolinium or contrast administration – Symmetrical involvement is unusual – Histologic confirmation is necessary for differentiation

Selected References

Mafee MF et al. Optic nerve sheath meningiomas. Role of MR imaging. Radiol Clin North Am 1999; 37(1): 37–58

Saeed P et al. Optic nerve sheath meningiomas. Ophthalmology 2003; 110(10): 2019–2030

Turbin RE et al. Diagnosis and treatment of orbital optic nerve sheath meningioma. Cancer Control 2004; 11(5): 334–341

Definition

▶ **Epidemiology**
Comprises 1% of all NHL ● 10% of all orbital tumors are NHL ● 85% B-cell lymphomas, 15% T-cell lymphomas ● 75% systemic involvement, 25% localized orbital involvement.

▶ **Etiology, pathophysiology, pathogenesis**
Extranodal manifestation of malignant lymphoproliferative disease ● Hereditary lymphocytic defect or dysfunction.

Imaging Signs

▶ **Modality of choice**
Gadolinium-enhanced MRI.

▶ **CT findings**
Soft-tissue-attenuation mass with pushing margins ● Possible infiltration of the lacrimal gland and eye muscles (coronal reformations!).

▶ **MRI findings**
Isointense mass on T1- and T2-weighted images ● Intense enhancement after gadolinium administration.

▶ **Pathognomonic findings**
Mass with smooth pushing margins, usually located at an anterosuperior site ● Enhances after contrast administration.

Clinical Aspects

▶ **Typical presentation**
Gradual development of painless exophthalmos ● Pain due to bone erosion ● Diplopia.

▶ **Treatment options**
Local radiotherapy (stage IE) ● Systemic chemotherapy (e.g., CHOP) for disseminated disease.

▶ **Course and prognosis**
Localized involvement: 75–100% cure rate ● Less risk of systemic disease with conjunctival NHL than orbital NHL.

Differential Diagnosis

Reactive lymphatic hyperplasia	– May be indistinguishable from lymphoma
	– Histologic confirmation may be necessary
Orbital pseudotumor	– Pain
	– Diffuse or ill-defined margins
Plasmacytoma	– Osteolytic lesions
Histiocytosis	– Smooth osteolytic lesions

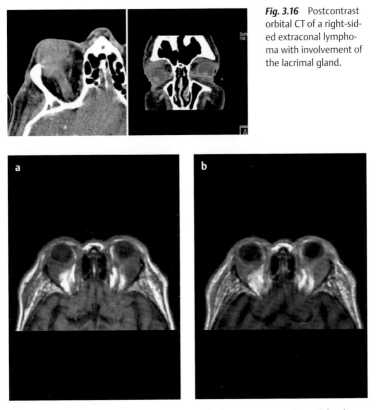

Fig. 3.16 Postcontrast orbital CT of a right-sided extraconal lymphoma with involvement of the lacrimal gland.

Fig. 3.17 a, b Bilateral intraorbital lymphomas. The lesions appear on T1-weighted images as hypointense masses (**a**) that enhance intensely after gadolinium administration (**b**).

Selected References

Coupland SE. Lymphoproliferative Läsionen der okulären Adnexe – Differenzialdiagnostische Leitlinien. Ophthalmologe 2004; 101(2): 197–215

Valvassori GE et al. Imaging of orbital lymphoproliferative disorders. Radiol Clin North Am 1999; 37(1): 135–150

Definition

▶ **Epidemiology**
Rarely diagnosed clinically (1–3%) • Usually diagnosed from pathohistology (10–37%) • A third of patients have no known primary tumor when the orbital metastasis is diagnosed.

▶ **Etiology, pathophysiology, pathogenesis**
Metastasis of malignant tumors to the orbit • Most common primary tumors: Breast cancer in women, lung cancer in men • Any malignant tumor may metastasize to the orbit (prostate, kidney, plasmacytoma, melanoma, etc.) • Head and neck tumors or metastases may directly invade the orbit (e.g., through the inferior orbital fissure).

Imaging Signs

▶ **Modality of choice**
CT, gadolinium-enhanced MRI.

▶ **CT findings**
Ill-defined, usually hyperdense mass • Intraocular (choroidal metastasis) or intraorbital location • Often distributed along the optic nerve, enhances after contrast administration • Bone destruction may occur.

▶ **MRI findings**
Isointense on T1-weighted images • Hyperintense on T2-weighted images • Enhances after gadolinium administration • T1-weighted with fat suppression useful for detecting diffusely infiltrating disease.

▶ **Pathognomonic findings**
Ill-defined intraocular or intraorbital mass.

Clinical Aspects

▶ **Typical presentation**
Mass • Exophthalmos • Pain • Visual impairment.

▶ **Treatment options**
Radiotherapy • Systemic chemotherapy • Surgical removal.

▶ **Course and prognosis**
Good prognosis with localized disease • Usually does not cause permanent visual impairment (60–80% response rate) • Signs of advanced tumor indicate a poor systemic prognosis (mean survival time with orbital metastasis is 6–17 months).

▶ **What does the clinician want to know?**
Diagnosis • Course.

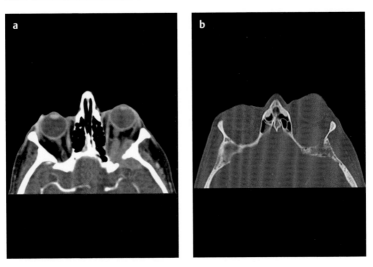

Fig. 3.18 a, b CT of left-sided apical orbital metastasis from known breast carcinoma, with extension through the superior orbital fissure into the anterior cranial fossa (**a**). Bone-window scan shows associated bone destruction in the posterosuperior orbital margin (**b**).

Differential Diagnosis

Orbital pseudotumor	– Acute pain – No bone destruction – Negative tumor history
Myositis	– Unilateral muscle thickening – No infiltration or bone destruction
Tolosa–Hunt syndrome	– Ophthalmoplegia – Granulomatous tissue in the orbital apex

Selected References

Chong VF et al. Radiology of the orbital apex. Australas Radiol 1999; 43(3): 294–302

Demirci H et al. Orbital tumors in the older adult population. Ophthalmology 2002; 109(2): 243–248

Dieing A et al. Orbital metastases in breast cancer: report of two cases and review of the literature. J Cancer Res Clin Oncol 2004; 130(12): 745–748

Lemke AJ et al. Differenzialdiagnostik intrakonaler orbitaler Raumforderungen unter Verwendung der hochauflösenden MRT mit Oberflächenspulen anhand von 78 Patienten. Fortschr. Röntgenstr 2004; 176(10): 1436–1446

McCaffery S et al. Three-dimensional high-resolution magnetic resonance imaging of ocular and orbital malignancies. Arch Ophthalmol 2002; 120(6): 747–754

Definition

▶ **Epidemiology**
  – *Deviated nasal septum:* Prevalence of 20–50% ● Usually asymptomatic.
  – *Pneumatization of one or more nasal turbinates ("concha bullosa"):* prevalence of 15–45%.
  – *Ethmoid cell variants:* infraorbital Haller cell (prevalence: 18–25%), Onodi cell (prevalence: 3–11%).
▶ **Etiology**
  Congenital or constitutional variants in the normal anatomy of the paranasal sinuses.

Imaging Signs

▶ **Modality of choice**
  CT (low-dose protocol) ● Replace direct coronal scans by coronal reformatting from a (multislice) spiral CT data set.
▶ **CT findings**
  Coronal scans or reformatted images:
  – Deviated nasal septum.
  – Pneumatization of nasal turbinates, particularly expansion of the middle turbinate ("concha bullosa").
  – Haller cell: Ethmoid cell located below the orbital floor, directly adjacent to the ostiomeatal unit.
  – Onodi cell: Posterior ethmoid cell extending above or close to the optic nerve canal (axial scans).
▶ **Selected normal values**
  No established norms for septal deviation.
  Evaluating the position of the cribriform plate in relation to the lateral part of the ethmoid roof (Keros classification):
  – Grade I: 1–3 mm.
  – Grade II: 4–7 mm.
  – Grade III: > 8 mm.

Clinical Aspects

▶ **Typical presentation**
  Usually asymptomatic, detected incidentally ● May affect physiologically important structures (e.g., development of chronic sinusitis due to narrowing of the ostiomeatal unit) ● Nasal airway obstruction (deviated septum).
▶ **Treatment options**
  Surgical correction of the nasal septum ● (Partial) removal of the nasal turbinates in functional sinus surgery.
▶ **Course and prognosis**
  Symptoms may persist in some cases despite corrective surgery.

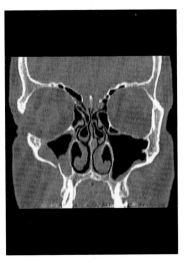

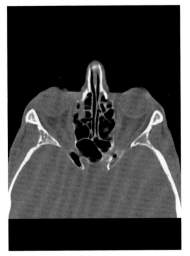

Fig. 4.1   Bilateral pneumatization of the middle turbinate ("concha bullosa"). On the left side, a Haller cell is typically positioned medially below the orbital floor, directly adjacent to the ostiomeatal unit. There is evidence of chronic sinusitis with slight mucosal swelling. The scan reveals a fracture in the right antral wall.

Fig. 4.2   Onodi cell on the right side shows typical extension into the superior clinoid process. It is closely related to the optic nerve canal.

▶ **What does the clinician want to know?**
Familiarity with anatomic details prior to functional sinus surgery can prevent intraoperative complications such as injuries to the anterior skull base, orbit, or optic nerve.

Tips and Pitfalls

Inaccurate assessment of the position of the ethmoid roof ● Poor visualization of Onodi cells in cranial MRI ● CT coverage should include the paranasal sinuses and facial skeleton.

Selected References
Bayram M et al. Important anatomic variations of the sinonasal anatomy in light of endoscopic surgery: a pictorial review. Eur Radiol 2001; 11(10): 1991–1997

Kösling S et al. Knöcherne Varianten im koronaren CT der Nasennebenhöhlen. Fortschr Röntgenstr 1993; 159(6): 506–510

Rao VM et al. Sinonasal imaging. Anatomy and pathology. Radiol Clin North Am 1998; 36(5): 921–39

Som PM, Curtin HD. Head and Neck Imaging. St. Louis: Mosby

Definition

▶ **Epidemiology**
Isolated fractures of the nasal bone account for 50% of all facial fractures ● The second most common type is the centrolateral midfacial fracture ● All subtypes have an approximately equal prevalence ● Fractures with displacement but no rotation are more common (30%) than fractures with a rotational component (6%) ● Orbital blowout fractures: 3–5% of all midfacial fractures.

▶ **Etiology, pathophysiology, pathogenesis**
Traumatic lesions of the facial skeleton caused by direct or indirect violence ● Sharp or blunt trauma that destroys the midfacial pillars (sagittal: vomer, lateral or medial antral and orbital walls, pterygoid processes; horizontal: orbital roof, orbital floor and zygomatic arch, maxilla).

Imaging Signs

▶ **Modality of choice**
CT (with coronal reformation).

▶ **CT findings**
Direct signs: Fracture lines ● Possible displacement of fragments.
Indirect signs: Air–fluid levels in the paranasal sinuses (hematosinus) ● Air collection in the soft tissues or cranial cavity ● Foreign body inclusion.
Classification:
– Nasal fractures.
– Central midfacial fractures (LeFort I–III).
– Lateral midfacial fractures (zygomatic arch fractures).
– Special type: blowout fracture of the orbital floor.

Clinical Aspects

▶ **Typical presentation**
Visible and palpable bony dehiscence, deviation, or depression ● Hematoma formation ● Nerve damage (infraorbital nerve damage occurs in 60–70% of LeFort II and III fractures) ● Visual impairment (e.g., diplopia).

▶ **Treatment options**
Fixation of fragments for primary fracture healing ● With complex fractures, separated portions of the midface can be reattached to the cranial base ● Nerve decompression.

▶ **Course and prognosis**
Early surgical treatment lowers the risk of osteomyelitis from 1.5% to 0.5% ● Posttraumatic sinusitis develops in up to 10% of cases.

▶ **What does the clinician want to know?**
Pattern of the fracture lines ● Classification by medial or centrolateral fracture type ● Presence of complications or involvement of adjacent structures (e.g., cranial cavity, orbit).

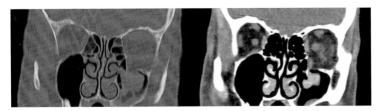

Fig. 4.3 Left orbital blowout fracture in a 42-year-old man. There are displaced bone fragments with herniation of orbital fat into the maxillary sinus.

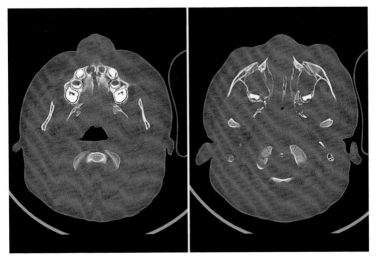

Fig. 4.4 Bilateral centrolateral midfacial fracture with involvement of the maxilla, maxillary sinus wall, and both pterygoid processes (LeFort type III), sustained in a bicycle accident.

Differential Diagnosis

Congenital lesions, e.g., encephalocele	– Altered anatomy with intact bony structures and no direct fracture signs
Posttherapeutic changes	– Absence of clinical symptoms – History – Defects with smooth margins – No malalignment or deformity
Cranial suture, osseous suture	– Side-to-side comparison – A "clear" air-filled sinus excludes a fracture of the sinus walls

Tips and Pitfalls

Avoid underestimating the severity of orbital floor injuries. Even without bone dehiscence, indirect signs such as fat herniation into the maxillary sinus or orbital air inclusions will confirm a blowout fracture.

Selected References

Hopper RA et al. Diagnosis of midfacial fractures with CT: what the surgeon needs to know. Radiographics 2006; 26: 783–793

Liman KF et al. Imaging of high-energy midfacial trauma: what the surgeon needs to know. Eur J Radiol 2003; 48: 17–32

Rhea JT et al. Helical CT and three-dimensional CT of facial and orbital injury. Radiol Clin North Am 1999; 37(3): 489–513

Turetschek K et al. Trauma des Gesichtsschädels und der Schädelkalotte. Radiologe 1998; 38(8): 659–666

Definition

▶ **Epidemiology**

Acute sinusitis is a common disease with rapid resolution ● It is usually a noso-comial infectious disease ● Approximately 20% of cases are secondary (e.g., to an odontogenic focus) ● Imaging studies are rarely necessary (3–5%, e.g., intraorbital spread) ● Approximately 5% of cases progress to chronic sinusitis ● Chronic sinusitis is more common in patients with predisposing factors (20% in cystic fibrosis, 30% in asthma).

▶ **Etiology, pathophysiology, pathogenesis**

Acute reaction of the nasal or sinus mucosa to inflammatory irritants ● Persistence longer than 3 months indicates chronic sinusitis.

Pathogenesis: May begin with nasal polyposis, for example (nonneoplastic circumscribed "polypoid" mucosal swelling) ● Swollen mucosa may obstruct the excretory ducts (e.g., ostiomeatal unit, frontal recess), causing retention of intraluminal secretions ● Local hypoxia promotes bacterial superinfection ● Submucous retention ("retention cysts") may result from the obstruction of mucinous gland secretions ● Leukocyte infiltration in response to recurrent irritation leads to chronic mucosal hypertrophy with polyp formation.

Imaging Signs

▶ **Modality of choice**

CT (low-dose protocol) ● Replace direct coronal scans by coronal reformations from a (multislice) spiral CT data set.

▶ **CT and MRI findings**

Circumferential mucosal swelling in paranasal sinuses ● Rounded, nonenhancing intrasinus masses that show no secondary signs of malignancy ● Chronic irritation leads to progressive thickening of the antral walls with luminal narrowing.

Orbital complications: Chandler stages:
– Stage I: Preseptal cellulitis.
– Stage II: Periostitis of the lamina papyracea, intraorbital cellulitis.
– Stage III: Subperiosteal abscess.
– Stage IV: Intraconal abscess.
– Stage V: Cavernous sinus thrombosis.

▶ **Selected measurement values**

Normal thickness of the nasal mucosa is 3 mm or less ● Typical circadian variations in the thickness of the turbinate mucosa ● Thickened mucosa: 5 mm = mild, 5–10 mm = moderate, > 10 mm = significant.

▶ **Pathognomonic findings**

Air–fluid level ● Submucosal retention of secretions (contrast-enhancing mucosa includes hypodense secretions).

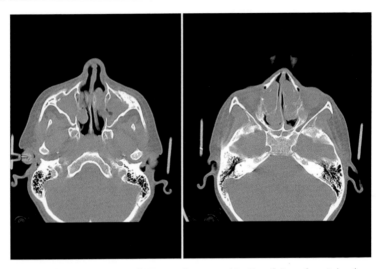

Fig. 4.5 Chronic sinusitis. Axial CT scans show a combination of circumferential and homogeneous opacity of the paranasal sinuses.

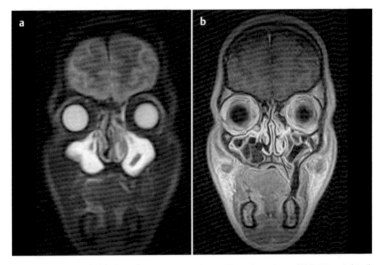

Fig. 4.6 a, b Rounded bulge of mucosa in each maxillary sinus shows high T2-weighted signal intensity (**a**). Mucosa enhancing after contrast administration over a focus of submucous retention is typical of a retention cyst (**b**, postgadolinium T1-weighted image).

Clinical Aspects

▶ **Typical presentation**
Mucous and purulent nasal discharge • Headache • Feeling of pressure • Nasal speech.

▶ **Treatment options**
Symptomatic treatment for acute (viral) sinusitis • Treatment of choice for chronic sinusitis or nasal polyposis: Reopen the ostiomeatal unit • Reestablish normal drainage by FESS (e.g., removal of the uncinate process and expansion of the infundibulum).

▶ **Course and prognosis**
Good prognosis for acute sinusitis with symptomatic treatment • Persistent (chronic) sinusitis or polyposis treated by FESS has an 80–90% clinical success rate • The recurrence rates for sinusitis and especially polyposis may range up to 30%, depending on predisposing factors.

▶ **What does the clinician want to know?**
Extent of the disease • Presence of normal anatomic variants • Complications (e.g., orbital involvement).

Differential Diagnosis

Sinus opacification due to neoplasia	– Frequently associated with bone destruction (especially by carcinoma) – Lymphomas show moderate contrast enhancement
Wegener granulomatosis	– Frequent septal destruction
Mycotic sinusitis	– Radiographically dense areas centrally within the mucus

Tips and Pitfalls

Limiting CT scans to a soft-tissue window may cause sinuses to appear clear and aerated • A "sinus" window (e.g., WW 1500) should always be used.

Selected References

Eggesbo HB et al. Radiological imaging of inflammatory lesions in the nasal cavity and paranasal sinuses. Eur Radiol 2006; 16: 872–888

Eustis HS et al. MR imaging and CT of orbital infections and complications in acute rhino-sinusitis. Radiol Clin North Am 1998; 36(6): 1165–1183

Vogl TJ et al. Chronische Infektionen der Nasennebenhöhlen. Radiologe 2000; 40(6): 500–506

Definition

▶ **Epidemiology**
Recurrent sinusitis: 10–20% ● Postoperative complications are rare (0.5–9%).

▶ **Etiology, pathophysiology, pathogenesis**
Intraoperative injury to neighbour structures ● Organ injury or intracranial lesion ● Rare: Hemorrhage, optic nerve injury, CSF fistula ● Less serious complications: Soft-tissue emphysema, hematoma, transient olfactory disturbance.

Imaging Signs

▶ **Modality of choice**
CT (low-dose protocol) ● Replace direct coronal scans by coronal reformations from a (multislice) spiral CT data set.

▶ **CT and MRI findings**
Demonstrate and describe anatomic structures that have been surgically altered or removed:
  – Frontal recess (persistent obstruction).
  – Ostiomeatal unit (obstruction or incomplete removal of uncinate process).
  – Lamina papyracea (dehiscence).
  – Cribriform plate, ethmoid roof (dehiscence).
  – Sphenoid sinus (dehiscence, cephalocele, optic nerve canal).
One or more of the following changes are found in typical cases:
  – Circumscribed expansion of the infundibulum due to removal of the uncinate process.
  – (Partial) removal of the middle nasal turbinate.
  – Ethmoidectomy.

▶ **Pathognomonic findings**
Expanded ostiomeatal unit ● Loss of individual bony lamellae in the ethmoid labyrinth ● Shortened and rounded middle turbinate.

Clinical Aspects

▶ **Typical presentation**
Many complications are diagnosed and treated in the early postoperative period (e.g., bleeding, infection, nerve injury) ● A smaller percentage of complications are manifested later (e.g., CSF fistula).

▶ **Treatment options**
Recurrent polyposis requires reoperation (e.g., for removal of polyps or scarred mucosa).

▶ **Course and prognosis**
Recurrence of sinusitis depends on anatomical factors (e.g., persistent septal deviation, residual ethmoid cells or anatomic variants) and predisposing factors (e.g., smoking, allergic disposition, asthma, cystic fibrosis).

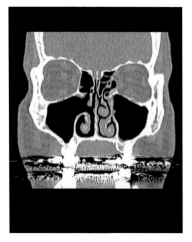

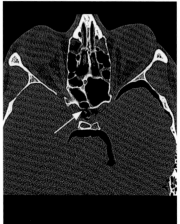

Fig. 4.7   Normal postoperative findings after surgical widening of the right ostio-meatal unit (FESS, coronal image reformatted from axial CT).

Fig. 4.8   Postoperative complication. Free intracranial air due to perforation of the sphenoid sinus (axial CT, arrow).

▶ **What does the clinician want to know?**

Evidence of intracranial or orbital complications • Normal postoperative status with no signs of recurrent polyposis • Causes of recurrence.

Differential Diagnosis

Posttraumatic lesions
  – History
  – Sites of irregular bone dehiscence

Tips and Pitfalls

A common error is to limit the evaluation to axial scans only.

Selected References

Ludwick JJ et al. A computed tomographic guide to endoscopic sinus surgery: axial and coronal views. J Comput Assist Tomogr 2002; 26(2): 317–322

Pockler C et al. CT der Nasennebenhöhlen vor endonasaler Chirurgie. Radiologe 1994; 34(2): 79–83

Sohaib SA. The effect of decreasing mAs on image quality and patient dose in sinus CT. Br J Radiol 2001; 74(878): 157–161

Som PM, Curtin HD. Head and Neck Imaging. St. Louis: Mosby; 2003

Younis RT et al. Intracranial complications of sinusitis: a 15-year review of 39 cases. Ear Nose Throat J 2002; 81(9): 636–638, 640–642, 644

Definition

▶ **Epidemiology**
Accounts for 4–6% of all polyps ● Allergic predisposition in 15–40% of patients.
▶ **Etiology, pathophysiology, pathogenesis**
True mucosal polyp of the maxillary sinus ● Extends into the nasal cavity through the infundibulum ● May extend into the choana.
Predisposing factors: Allergic predisposition ● Infectious rhinosinusitis ● Diabetes mellitus ● Cystic fibrosis ● Aspirin intolerance.

Imaging Signs

▶ **Modality of choice**
CT (with coronal reformations).
▶ **CT findings**
Well-circumscribed mass of soft-tissue density ● Extends from the maxillary sinus into the nasal cavity ● May extend into the nasopharynx.
▶ **MRI findings**
Mass with high T2-weighted signal intensity ● Low T1-weighted signal intensity ● Does not enhance after gadolinium administration.
▶ **Pathognomonic findings**
Polyp that extends into the nasal cavity and may enter the choana.

Clinical Aspects

▶ **Typical presentation**
Unilateral nasal airway obstruction ● Pain in rare cases ● Adolescent patient.
▶ **Treatment options**
Resection of polyps ● Desensitization is advised in patients with an allergic predisposition.
▶ **Course and prognosis**
Good prognosis following complete removal ● Recurrence rate approximately 20–30%.
▶ **What does the clinician want to know?**
Diagnosis ● Extent ● Additional manifestations of chronic sinusitis, if present ● Preoperative anatomic variants.

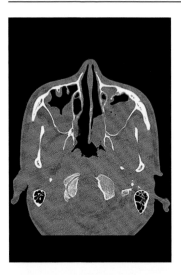

Fig. 4.9 Choanal polyp extending from the left maxillary sinus into the nasal cavity. Bilateral chronic sinusitis.

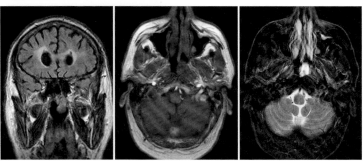

Fig. 4.10 Choanal polyp on the left side extending into the nasopharynx (FLAIR and T1-weighted: intermediate signal intensity; T2-weighted: high signal intensity).

Differential Diagnosis

Juvenile nasopharyngeal angiofibroma	– History – Very vascular, enhancing lesion extending into the pterygopalatine fossa – Rare involvement of the maxillary sinus
Encephalocele	– Nasal mass extending from the cranial cavity – Bone defect or developmental anomaly
Nasopharyngeal carcinoma	– Usually spares the paranasal sinuses – Destructive lesion with other signs of malignancy (e.g., lymph node metastases)

Tips and Pitfalls

Classic presentation with bell-shaped extension is best appreciated on the primary axial image.

Selected References

Chung SK et al. Surgical, radiologic, and histologic findings of the antrochoanal polyp. Am J Rhinol 2002; 16(2): 71–76

Definition

▶ **Epidemiology**
Two-thirds of all mucoceles occur in the frontal sinus • Other sites: ethmoid cells (20–25%), maxillary sinuses (5–10%), sphenoid sinus (5–10%).

▶ **Etiology, pathophysiology, pathogenesis**
Paranasal sinus mass caused by retained secretions • Associated bone remodeling • Sinus obstruction (inflammatory, posttraumatic, postoperative) leading to retention of secretions • Constant pressure causes gradual expansion and thinning of the bony sinus walls.

Imaging Signs

▶ **Modality of choice**
CT • Reformations in multiple planes • Postcontrast scans to evaluate intracranial involvement.

▶ **CT findings**
Well-circumscribed mass causing smooth contour changes • Originates from the paranasal sinuses • Expansion of bony boundaries • Extension into adjacent structures • Compresses adjacent structures without causing destructive changes • Pyocele shows increased attenuation values (purulent secretions) and air inclusions.

▶ **MRI findings**
Rounded mass with high T2-weighted signal intensity • Inspissation of secretions leads to reversal of signal pattern (low T2-weighted signal intensity, high T1-weighted signal intensity) • Unlike slow-growing tumors, does not enhance after gadolinium administration.

▶ **Pathognomonic findings**
Well-circumscribed mass with associated thinning and expansion of bony sinus walls, does not enhance after contrast administration.

Clinical Aspects

▶ **Typical presentation**
Usually asymptomatic • Pain in rare cases • Compression effects can cause numerous clinical symptoms such as proptosis (frontal or ethmoid sinus), unilateral visual impairment (ethmoid or sphenoid sinus), and nasal airway obstruction (maxillary sinus).

▶ **Treatment options**
Surgical removal of the mucocele.

▶ **Course and prognosis**
Should not recur after complete removal, even through an endonasal approach • Cranial nerve symptoms may regress, depending on the lesion duration • Complication: Pyocele development due to bacterial superinfection (painful).

▶ **What does the clinician want to know?**
Diagnosis • Location and extent • Relationship to other structures • Complications.

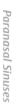
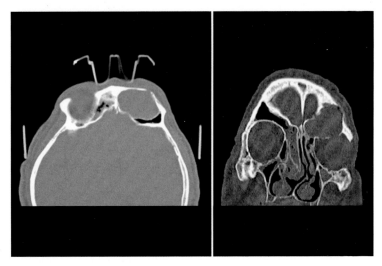

Fig. 4.11 Typical frontal sinus mucocele. A mass of fluid attenuation has caused a rounded bulge in the bony sinus wall with upward displacement of the eyeball.

Differential Diagnosis

Benign sinus tumors (e.g., papilloma)	– Usually causes less uniform bone remodeling – Contrast-enhancing tumor tissue
Choanal polyp	– Does not cause sinus expansion, but extends into the nasal cavity
Odontogenic cyst	– Rounded mass on the floor of the maxillary sinus, does not cause sinus expansion – Usually contains detectable root material

Tips and Pitfalls

A large mass may be mistaken for a tumor ● Be sure to evaluate adjacent structures ● Contrast administration aids in identifying a neoplastic process and complications.

Selected References

Har-El G. Endoscopic management of 108 sinus mucoceles. Laryngoscope 2001; 111(12): 2131–2134

Lloyd G et al. Optimum imaging for mucoceles. J Laryngol Otol 2000; 114(3): 233–236

Serrano E et al. Surgical management of paranasal sinus mucoceles: a long-term study of 60 cases. Otolaryngol Head Neck Surg 2004; 131(1): 133–140

Som PM, Curtin HD. Head and Neck Imaging. St. Louis: Mosby

Definition

▶ **Epidemiology**
A fungal etiology is present in 6–8% of all chronic sinusitis cases.

▶ **Etiology, pathophysiology, pathogenesis**
Sinusitis resulting from a mycotic infection, usually with *Aspergillus* species •
Four forms are distinguished by their course:
– Form I: Acute invasive.
– Form II: Chronic invasive.
– Form III: Mycetoma.
– Form IV: Allergic fungal sinusitis.
Acute invasive forms are most common in immunocompromised patients (often mucormycosis species, especially in diabetes mellitus, HIV, and leukopenic patients) • Noninvasive forms occur in immunocompetent patients with chronic sinusitis or an allergic disposition.

Imaging Signs

▶ **Modality of choice**
Contrast-enhanced CT, gadolinium-enhanced MRI.

▶ **CT findings**
Complete opacification of one or more sinuses without a fluid level • Allergic fungal sinusitis is indistinguishable from chronic sinusitis with multiple polyps
• Central hyperdensity (metabolic products, displaced root filling) may be seen
• Acute invasive form: bone-destructive lesions and infiltrating, invasive spread into surrounding structures (orbit, skull base, cranial interior).

▶ **MRI findings**
High T2-weighted signal intensity, low T1-weighted signal intensity • Does not enhance after gadolinium administration • Acute invasive form: infiltrating, destructive expansion outside the sinus, best appreciated in T1-weighted and fat-suppressed sequences after gadolinium injection.

▶ **Pathognomonic findings**
Central hyperdensity on CT in allergic fungal sinusitis and infections with a mycetoma • Frequent bilateral involvement of multiple sinuses • Mass thins the bony walls or may cause irregular focal demineralization • Invasive form may cause bone destruction • Diffuse infiltration of surrounding structures by invasive fungal sinusitis.

Clinical Aspects

▶ **Typical presentation**
Acute invasive form: Severe clinical manifestations • Fever • Lethargy ranging to coma • Frequent visual impairment due to orbital complications • Intracranial extension with associated neurological symptoms.
Noninvasive forms: May be asymptomatic • May produce symptoms of chronic sinusitis.

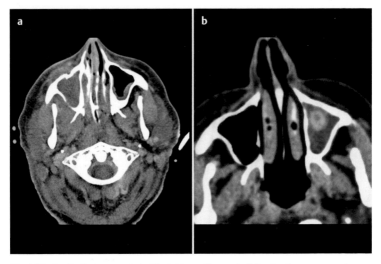

Fig. 4.12 a, b Patient presented with right maxillary pain following bone marrow transplantation for acute myeloid leukemia. CT shows acute invasive *Aspergillus* sinusitis with infiltration of the facial soft tissues and infratemporal fossa, predominantly on the right side (**a**). The chronic form (**b**) shows increased central density.

▸ **Treatment options**
Acute invasive form requires prompt, complete surgical eradication, which may include resection of involved adjacent structures (e.g., orbit) ● Concomitant antimycotic agents (e.g., amphotericin B, caspofungin) ● Treatment of chronic forms is basically similar but less radical and urgent.

▸ **Course and prognosis**
If diagnosis or treatment is delayed, acute invasive mucormycosis is fatal in up to 40% of cases ● Chronic forms have a markedly better prognosis and may resolve completely after surgery.

▸ **What does the clinician want to know?**
Diagnosis ● Extent ● Involvement of adjacent structures by invasive forms.

Differential Diagnosis

Malignant tumor	– History, course
	– Tumors show more intense enhancement after contrast administration
Chronic sinusitis	– Indistinguishable from allergic fungal sinusitis by imaging alone (sinobronchial syndrome)

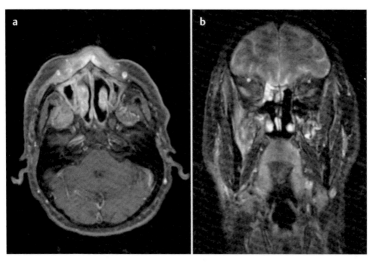

Fig. 4.13 a, b A 65-year-old woman with diabetes mellitus. Mucormycosis of the right maxillary sinus developed secondary to an odontogenic abscess, leading to trigeminal and facial nerve palsies. MRI shows diffuse spread of inflammation into the infratemporal fossa. Fat-suppressed T1-weighted image after gadolinium administration (**a**) and T2-weighted image with fat suppression (**b**).

Tips and Pitfalls

Always consider the possibility of invasive mycosis, especially in people with diabetes and immunocompromised patients • Diagnosis should be established promptly, by biopsy if necessary, to allow early initiation of therapy.

Selected References

Bent JP et al. Diagnosis of allergic fungal sinusitis. Otolaryngol Head Neck Surg 1994; 111(5): 580–588

Eggesbo HB. Radiological imaging of inflammatory lesions in the nasal cavity and paranasal sinuses. Eur Radiol 2006; 16: 872–888

Morpeth JF et al. Fungal sinusitis: an update. Ann Allergy Asthma Immunol 1996; 76(2): 128–139

Mukherji SK et al. Allergic fungal sinusitis: CT findings. Radiology 1998; 207(2): 417–422

4 Wegener Granulomatosis

Definition

▶ **Epidemiology**
Nasal cavity and paranasal sinuses affected in 60–70% of cases • More than 90% of patients have pulmonary involvement.

▶ **Etiology, pathophysiology, pathogenesis**
Idiopathic, necrotizing, granulomatous vasculitis of the upper respiratory tract • Renal involvement in some cases • Etiology uncertain • Development of noncaseating granulomas or inflammatory reactions.

Imaging Signs

▶ **Modality of choice**
CT (to detect bone destruction) • Gadolinium-enhanced MRI.

▶ **CT findings**
Rounded lesion of soft-tissue density • Frequently located in the midline • Opacification of the nasal cavity and paranasal sinuses • Some cases show "moth-eaten" bone destruction initially affecting the septum and later involving the medial antral walls and turbinates.

▶ **MRI findings**
Nodular masses in the mucosa • Usually show high T2-weighted signal intensity • Inhomogeneous enhancement after gadolinium administration.

▶ **Pathognomonic findings**
Mass located near the midline • Shows enhancement after contrast administration and bone destruction.

Clinical Aspects

▶ **Typical presentation**
Often misinterpreted as chronic sinusitis for some years • Purulent nasal discharge • Epistaxis • Pain.

▶ **Treatment options**
Immunosuppression (e.g., steroids, cyclophosphamide) • Surgical eradication may be tried, especially in patients with orbital complications.

▶ **Course and prognosis**
Disease confined to the paranasal sinuses without systemic involvement often takes a benign course • Possible destruction of midfacial structures with intracranial extension.

▶ **What does the clinician want to know?**
Presumptive diagnosis • Definitive diagnosis requires histologic confirmation • Extent of disease • Bone destruction.

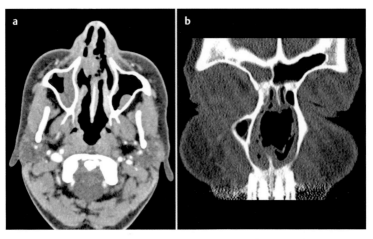

Fig. 4.14 a, b   Wegener granulomatosis. CT scans show a midline mass of soft-tissue density in the nasal cavity (**a**) that has eroded the nasal septum (**b**). Initial finding in a patient with clinical complaints mainly involving the head.

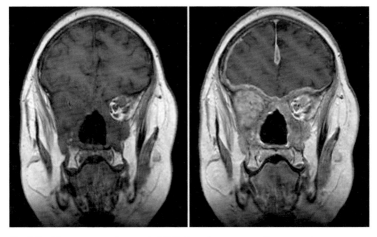

Fig. 4.15   Wegener granulomatosis (MRI) after sinus surgery. Contrast enhancement of the soft tissue signifies intraorbital and intracranial extension of the granulomatous process.

Differential Diagnosis

NHL	– May show more intense enhancement
	– Otherwise, lesions near the midline may be indistinguishable by their imaging features
Invasive fungal sinusitis	– History and course
Toxic (e.g., "cocaine nose")	– History
	– Bone destruction with relatively smooth margins
	– Scant granulomatous tissue

Tips and Pitfalls

Always consider the disease in the differential diagnosis • Avoid missing spread past sinus boundaries.

Selected References

Benoudiba F et al. Sinonasal Wegener's granulomatosis: CT characteristics. Neuroradiology 2003; 45(2): 95–99

Borges A et al. Midline destructive lesions of the sinonasal tract: simplified terminology based on histopathologic criteria. AJNR Am J Neuroradiol 2000; 21(2): 331–336

Muhle C et al. MRI of the nasal cavity, the paranasal sinuses and orbits in Wegener's granulomatosis. Eur Radiol 1997; 7(4): 566–570

Shin MS et al. Wegener's granulomatosis upper respiratory tract and pulmonary radiographic manifestations in 30 cases with pathogenetic consideration. Clin Imaging 1998; 22(2): 99–104

Definition

▶ **Epidemiology**
Peak occurrence between 14 and 17 years of age ● Affects young males almost exclusively.

▶ **Etiology, pathophysiology, pathogenesis**
Benign, locally invasive, vascular tumor in teenage males ● Most common benign tumor of the nasopharynx ● 5–20% extend to the skull base, with possible intracranial spread through the neuroforamina.

Imaging Signs

▶ **Modality of choice**
Contrast-enhanced CT, gadolinium-enhanced MRI, MRA.

▶ **CT findings**
Intensely enhancing tumor ● Grows from the sphenopalatine foramen into the pterygopalatine fossa, pterygoid fossa, middle cranial fossa, and maxillary sinus.

▶ **MRI findings**
Intermediate T2-weighted signal intensity ● Low T1-weighted signal intensity with intense enhancement after gadolinium administration ● MRA may show hypertrophy of the maxillary artery or ascending pharyngeal artery ● Perfusion measurements show a dropout effect (arterial perfusion) ● T2-weighted imaging shows linear or punctate hypointensity (flow voids in hypertrophic vessels).

▶ **Pathognomonic findings**
Intensely enhancing tumor arising from the pterygopalatine fossa in teenage males.

Clinical Aspects

▶ **Typical presentation**
Nasal airway obstruction, usually unilateral ● Epistaxis ● Pain.

▶ **Treatment options**
Treatment of choice is surgical removal ● Preoperative embolization may be helpful to reduce intraoperative blood loss, depending on tumor size ● Another option is radiotherapy—primary and for recurrence.

▶ **Course and prognosis**
Benign tumor has a 15–25% local recurrence rate after surgery indicated by space-occupying lesion with intense enhancement after contrast administration ● Recurrence may be managed by resection or radiotherapy ● Recurrences are less common after radiotherapy ● Cataract or CNS radiation injuries may occur.

▶ **What does the clinician want to know?**
Extent ● Possible need for preoperative transcatheter embolization.

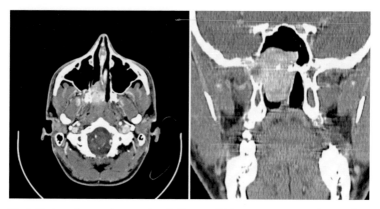

Fig. 4.16   Juvenile nasopharyngeal angiofibroma. CT demonstrates a typical intensely enhancing tumor arising from the pterygopalatine fossa and extending into the nasal cavity.

Differential Diagnosis

Choanal polyp	– Nonenhancing
	– Endonasal mass without extension into the pterygopalatine fossa
Malignant tumors	– Usually originates in the sinuses
(e.g., rhabdomyosarcoma)	– Pterygopalatine fossa is usually not affected
	– Younger patients
	– Homogeneous, intensely enhancing mass (no flow voids)

Tips and Pitfalls

Coronal MR images or reformatted coronal CT images are essential for evaluating intracranial extension.

Selected References

Chagnaud C et al. Postoperative follow-up of juvenile nasopharyngeal angiofibromas: assessment by CT scan and MR imaging. Eur Radiol 1998; 8(5): 756–764

Scholtz AW et al. Juvenile nasopharyngeal angiofibroma: management and therapy. Laryngoscope 2001; 111(4 Pt 1): 681–687

Sennes LU et al. Juvenile nasopharyngeal angiofibroma: the routes of invasion. Rhinology 2003; 41(4): 235–240

Turowski B et al. Interventional neuroradiology of the head and neck. Neuroimaging Clin N Am 2003; 13(3): 619–645

Definition

▶ **Epidemiology**
Papillomas comprise 0.5–5% of all tumors of the nose and paranasal sinuses ●
75% are inverted papillomas ● Male predominance with peak occurrence in the
fourth to seventh decades ● 3–24% progress to carcinoma (mainly squamous cell
carcinoma).

▶ **Etiology, pathophysiology, pathogenesis**
Epithelial tumor ● Arises from lateral nasal wall ● Extends into paranasal sinuses
(usually the maxillary sinus) ● Etiology uncertain ● Association with human
papillomavirus ● Fungiform papillomas develop on the nasal septum.

Imaging Signs

▶ **Modality of choice**
CT, gadolinium-enhanced MRI.

▶ **CT findings**
Unilateral tumor of soft-tissue density ● Arises from the lateral nasal wall ● Lobulated surface ● Serpentine enhancement of infolded mucosa after contrast administration ● Intratumoral calcifications possible ● Slow-growing tumors may
cause bone erosion.

▶ **MRI findings**
Low T1-weighted signal intensity and moderately high T2-weighted signal intensity ● T2-weighting shows irregular signal pattern that is well demarcated
after gadolinium administration (as in CT) ● Central necrosis or infiltration of
surrounding structures are likely signs of malignant transformation.

▶ **Pathognomonic findings**
Tumor of soft-tissue density at the level of the middle nasal turbinate ● Obstruction of ostiomeatal unit leads to opacification of frontal and maxillary sinus and
anterior ethmoid cells ● Typical serpentine enhancement pattern on CT and MRI
after contrast/gadolinium administration.

Clinical Aspects

▶ **Typical presentation**
Sinusitis due to obstruction of ostiomeatal unit ● Nasal speech ● Epistaxis.

▶ **Treatment options**
Complete surgical removal ● Besides the classic maxillectomy approach, endoscopic techniques are increasingly used.

▶ **Course and prognosis**
High recurrence rate, especially with classic operative techniques ● Lower recurrence rate with endoscopic techniques (15–20%).

▶ **What does the clinician want to know?**
Diagnosis ● Extent ● Possible signs of malignancy.

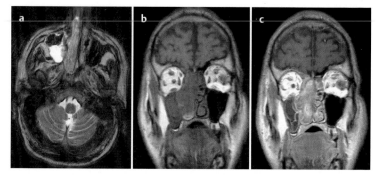

Fig. 4.17 a–c Tumor of soft-tissue density arising from the lateral nasal wall without signs of malignancy. Mucus retention is noted in the right maxillary sinus (inhomogeneous T2-weighted signal intensity, **a**). Plain T1-weighted image (**b**). Gadolinium produces an intense, somewhat whorled pattern of enhancement (**c**).

Differential Diagnosis

Retention cyst	– Nonenhancing mass with smooth margins
Choanal polyp	– Rounded polyp arising from the maxillary sinus, does not show significant contrast enhancement
Nasopharyngeal angiofibroma	– Younger patients – Originates in the nasopharynx and involves the pterygopalatine fossa
Malignant tumors (e.g., squamous cell carcinoma)	– Inhomogeneous enhancement – Direct signs of malignancy – Occasionally indistinguishable from papilloma

Tips and Pitfalls

Look for possible signs of malignancy (infiltration, bone destruction, necrosis) • Locate site of origin and assess enhancement pattern to differentiate it from other masses.

Selected References

Dammann F et al. Inverted papilloma of the nasal cavity and the paranasal sinuses: using CT for primary diagnosis and follow-up. AJR Am J Roentgenol 1999; 172(2): 543–548

Kaufman MR et al. Sinonasal papillomas: clinicopathologic review of 40 patients with inverted and oncocytic schneiderian papillomas. Laryngoscope 2002; 112(8 Pt 1): 1372–1377

Ojiri H et al. Potentially distinctive features of sinonasal inverted papilloma on MR imaging. AJR Am J Roentgenol 2000; 175(2): 465–468

Definition

▶ **Epidemiology**
Prevalence of 1:100 000 • Most common in older males • 3 % of all head and neck tumors are carcinomas • Most common types are squamous cell carcinoma (50 %), undifferentiated carcinoma (20 %), adenoid cystic carcinoma and adeno-carcinoma (10 % each) • *Sites of predilection:* maxillary sinus antrum (50–60 %), ethmoid cells (10–25 %), and nasal cavity (15–30 %).

▶ **Etiology, pathophysiology, pathogenesis**
Malignant epithelial tumor • Arises from the mucosa or small mucous glands • Risk is increased by prolonged exposure to exogenous toxins (e.g., nickel, chromium, wood workers), with long latent period.

Imaging Signs

▶ **Modality of choice**
Gadolinium-enhanced MRI, contrast-enhanced CT.

▶ **CT findings**
Mass of soft-tissue density • Inhomogeneous enhancement (necrotic areas) • Bone destruction • Often infiltrates surrounding structures.

▶ **MRI findings**
Intermediate signal intensity on T1- and T2-weighted images • Mass that enhances after gadolinium administration • Central sparing due to necrosis • Perineural tumor spread can be detected in fat-suppressed sequences and by multiplanar imaging • Retained secretions often show high T2-weighted signal intensity • Chronic retention may show decreased T2-weighted signal intensity due to inspissation of the contents.
  – T1: Tumor confined to paranasal sinus, no bone destruction.
  – T2: Anterior and/or posterior bone destruction (buccal soft tissues, maxilla).
  – T3: Posterior and/or superior bone destruction (posterior wall of maxillary sinus, orbital floor, pterygoid processes, anterior ethmoid cells).
  – T4: Extension into the orbit, cranial cavity, nasopharynx, pterygopalatine fossa, soft palate, clivus, posterior ethmoid cells.

▶ **Pathognomonic findings**
Unilateral, bone-destructive, enhancing tumor usually located in the maxillary sinus antrum, nasal cavity, or anterior ethmoid cells • Perineural tumor spread.

Clinical Aspects

▶ **Typical presentation**
Headache, sinus pain • Sinusitis • Visual impairment • Tooth loss.

▶ **Treatment options**
Radical excision and radiotherapy • Chemotherapy • Possible multimodal therapy.

▶ **Course and prognosis**
High local recurrence rate (20–50 %), 80 % during the first year • 5-year survival rate of 60–75 % • T1 tumors have a 100 % survival rate with appropriate treatment.

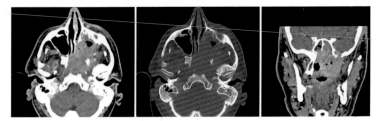

Fig. 4.18   T4 squamous cell carcinoma of the left maxillary sinus. MR image shows an inhomogeneously enhancing soft-tissue mass with associated bone destruction and infiltration of the nasopharynx, infratemporal fossa, and skull base (reformatted coronal image).

► **What does the clinician want to know?**

Diagnosis (differentiation from sinusitis) ● Extent of tumor ● Infiltration of surrounding tissues or bone erosion ● Skull base involvement or perineural spread ● *Landmarks:* buccal soft tissues, pterygopalatine fossa, orbit, maxilla, neuroforamina.

Differential Diagnosis

Invasive fungal sinusitis	– Often indistinguishable from carcinoma – Brief history
Wegener granulomatosis	– Midline lesion that does not show significant enhancement after contrast administration – Bone destruction and infiltrative growth may be indistinguishable from carcinoma in some cases
NHL	– Minimal enhancement – Bone erosion is more typical than bone destruction

Tips and Pitfalls

May be misinterpreted as chronic sinusitis ● Failure to visualize and evaluate perineural infiltration.

Selected References

Caldemeyer KS et al. Imaging features and clinical significance of perineural spread or extension of head and neck tumors. Radiographics 1998; 18(1): 97–110

Goldenberg D et al. Malignant tumors of the nose and paranasal sinuses: a retrospective review of 291 cases. Ear Nose Throat J 2001; 80(4): 272–277

Loerner LA et al. Imaging of neoplasms of the paranasal sinuses. Magn Reson Imaging Clin N Am 2002; 10: 467–493

Rao VM et al. Sinonasal imaging. Anatomy and pathology. Radiol Clin North Am 1998; 36(5): 921–939

Definition

▶ **Epidemiology**
Approximately 50% of NHL patients have head and neck involvement, usually of the cervical lymph nodes ● Extranodal disease is present in 10% ● Approximately equal prevalence of B- and T-cell types ● Sinus involvement by Hodgkin disease is much less common.

▶ **Etiology, pathophysiology, pathogenesis**
Extranodal involvement of the paranasal sinuses by NHL ● Etiology uncertain.

Imaging Signs

▶ **Modality of choice**
Contrast-enhanced CT, gadolinium-enhanced MRI.

▶ **CT findings**
Soft-tissue mass in the nose or paranasal sinuses, usually showing moderate, homogeneous enhancement ● May extend into the nasopharynx (Waldeyer ring) ● Cervical lymphadenopathy ● Bone erosion is more typical than bone destruction ● Imaging appearance may mimic carcinoma ● Necrotic areas and/or stippled calcifications may appear after treatment.

▶ **MRI findings**
Intermediate signal intensity on T1- and T2-weighted images ● Homogeneous enhancement of tumor mass after gadolinium administration ● Intracranial extension best appreciated in gadolinium-enhanced T1-weighted sequence with fat suppression.

▶ **Pathognomonic findings**
Lymphomas can mimic all benign and malignant entities (from nasal polyps and papillomas to carcinomas).

Clinical Aspects

▶ **Typical presentation**
Mass lesion ● Obstruction ● Sinusitis ● Occasional epistaxis.

▶ **Treatment options**
Chemotherapy and/or radiotherapy ● Initial biopsy of isolated lesion.

▶ **Course and prognosis**
Five-year survival rate 40–90%, depending on tumor stage.

▶ **What does the clinician want to know?**
Diagnosis ● Location (for biopsy) ● Involvement of basal brain structures or intracranial extension.

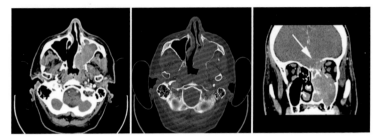

Fig. 4.19 NHL in a 62-year-old man. CT shows an enhancing mass of soft-tissue density extending from the left maxillary sinus into the pterygoid fossa and cranial cavity (arrow), with associated bone erosion.

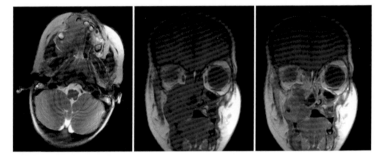

Fig. 4.20 NHL in a 3-year-old boy. MR image shows an enhancing soft-tissue mass in the right maxillary sinus that has infiltrated the facial soft tissues and orbit.

Differential Diagnosis

Nasal polyposis	– Nonenhancing
	– No bone erosion
Inverted papilloma	– No bone erosion
	– Serpentine enhancement pattern
Carcinoma	– Frequent, conspicuous bone destruction
	– Pressure erosion more likely with NHL
	– May have very similar imaging appearance in some cases

Tips and Pitfalls

Without contrast administration, NHL may be misinterpreted as chronic sinusitis or polyposis ● Look for bony changes and spread beyond sinus boundaries ● If findings are equivocal, biopsy should be done.

Selected References

Gufler H et al. MRI of lymphomas of the orbits and the paranasal sinuses. J Comput Assist Tomogr 1997; 21(6): 887–891

Nakamura K et al. Primary non-Hodgkin lymphoma of the sinonasal cavities: correlation of CT evaluation with clinical outcome. Radiology 1997; 204(2): 431–435

Weber AL et al. Hodgkin and non-Hodgkin lymphoma of the head and neck: clinical, pathologic, and imaging evaluation. Neuroimaging Clin N Am 2003; 13(3): 371–392

Definition

▶ **Epidemiology**

Most common congenital mass of the nasopharynx ● Incidence: 4% ● Peak occurrence at 15–60 years of age ● Usually an incidental finding, detected in 1–5% of cranial MR examinations.

▶ **Etiology, pathophysiology, pathogenesis**

Synonym: Pharyngeal bursa ● Benign cyst of the posterosuperior nasopharynx based on an embryogenic variant ● Midline cyst located in the submucous plane of the posterosuperior nasopharynx ● Usually results from inflammatory obstruction of a persistent embryonic communication between the primitive pharynx and notochord ● Usually asymptomatic ● Rarely undergoes abscess formation.

Imaging Signs

▶ **Modality of choice**

MRI.

▶ **CT findings**

Incidental finding ● Cyst located in the posterior midline of the nasopharynx ● Iso- or hyperdense to muscle ● Small cysts are difficult to diagnose ● As in MRI, lesion delineation is usually improved by contrast administration.

▶ **MRI findings**

Cyst shows intermediate to high T1-weighted signal intensity, depending on its protein content ● Cyst wall occasionally shows enhancement after gadolinium administration ● T2-weighted and STIR sequences usually show a uniformly hyperintense, benign cyst with well-defined margins.

▶ **Selected values**

Cyst from several millimeters to 3 cm in diameter ● Chronic inflammatory changes in cysts > 2 cm.

▶ **Pathognomonic findings**

Midline cyst with high T1-weighted and T2-weighted signal intensity located in the submucous plane of the posterior pharyngeal space.

Clinical Aspects

▶ **Typical presentation**

Over 99% are clinically silent ● Rarely causes eustachian tube compression, nasal speech, or abscess formation ● Rare cases show chronic infection with "Thornwaldt syndrome": Pharyngitis, halitosis, stiff neck, and occipital headache.

▶ **Treatment options**

Treatment is unnecessary in asymptomatic cases ● Antibiotic therapy ● Transoral excision or marsupialization for chronically infected or painful cysts.

▶ **Course and prognosis**

Cases detected incidentally do not require follow-up ● Operative treatment is curative.

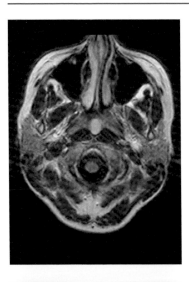

Fig. 5.1 Unenhanced T2-weighted MR image shows a Thornwaldt cyst located in the anterior midline between the bellies of the longus colli muscle in the roof of the nasopharynx. The cyst content is usually hyperintense on T2-weighted images.

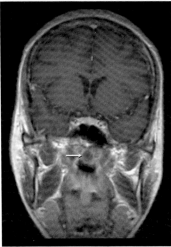

Fig. 5.2 T1-weighted image after gadolinium injection (same patient as in Fig. 5.**1**). Here the cyst contents appear iso- to hypointense to muscle. The hyperintense ring surrounding the cyst is composed of the cyst wall and enhancing pharyngeal mucosa after gadolinium administration (arrow).

Differential Diagnosis

Adenoid hyperplasia	– Diffuse, usually paramedian hyperplasia of lymphatic tissue – Permeated by enhancing bands
Adenoid retention cyst (mucosal cyst)	– Low T1-weighted signal intensity – Often located in the lateral recess – Multiple – Characteristic heart- or pear-shaped configuration
Choanal polyp	– Low T1-weighted signal intensity – Obstructs the nasopharyngeal space from the front
Rathke cleft cyst	– Incomplete embryonic occlusion of Rathke pouch – Caudal cyst, usually located in the sphenoid bone
Cephalocele	– May be found in the nasopharynx, but shows a definite communication with cerebral structures

Tips and Pitfalls

Cysts with a characteristic appearance on imaging are rarely misdiagnosed.

Selected References

Chong VF et al. Radiology of the nasopharynx: pictorial essay. Australas Radiol 2000; 44(1): 5–13

Ikushima I et al. MR Imaging of Tornwaldt's Cysts. AJR 1999; 172: 1663–1665

Weissman JL. Thornwaldt cysts. J Otolaryngol 1992; 13(6): 381–385

Definition

▶ **Epidemiology**
Disk space infection and vertebral body involvement are clinically indistinguish-able • Treatment for both conditions is the same (hence, spondylodiskitis is clin-ically synonymous with spondylitis, diskitis, and vertebral osteomyelitis) • Prev-alence ranges from 1:50 000 (Europe) to 11 % (Africa) • Risk is increased in diabetes, HIV infection, steroid use, and alcohol and drug misuse • 2:1 male-to-female ratio • Bimodal peak at 5–30 years and 50–60 years • Diskitis is more common in children younger than 3 years (better vascularity) • Vertebral osteomyelitis is more common in children over 7 years.

▶ **Etiology, pathophysiology, pathogenesis**
Inflammation of adjacent vertebral bodies and the associated disk • Usually spreads by the hematogenous route • Occasionally postoperative • Often leads to prevertebral, paravertebral or epidural abscess formation • Pediatric cases may result from streptococcal or *Bartonella henselae* infection and cat-scratch disease • Occasionally posttraumatic.

Imaging Signs

▶ **Modality of choice**
MRI (96 % sensitivity, 94 % accuracy) • CT if gas-forming organisms are suspect-ed • $^{99\,m}$Tc scanning can also be done to map disseminated disease.

▶ **MRI findings**
T1-weighted: Disk space narrowing • Adjacent hypointense endplates • Enhancement of disk space and vertebral bodies after gadolinium administra-tion • Associated perivertebral and epidural reaction or abscess (detection rate increased by enhancement after gadolinium administration on fat-suppressed T1-weighted images).
Postgadolinium T1-weighted: Intermediate signal intensity at discovertebral junctions • Increased signal intensity in the vertebral body.
T2-weighted, STIR: Increased signal intensity of disk and vertebral body.

▶ **Selected normal values**
Disk space heights: C2 < C3 < C4 < C5 < C6 ≥ C7 • Retropharyngeal space up to 7 mm at C2 level • Retrotracheal space up to 22 mm at C6 level.

▶ **Pathognomonic findings**
Disk space shows high T2-weighted signal intensity and enhances after gadolini-um administration on T1-weighted image.

Clinical Aspects

▶ **Typical presentation**
Diagnosis is often delayed due to nonspecific inflammatory signs (e.g., high CRP, fever, lethargy) • Local muscle guarding • Nuchal pain aggravated by move-ment • Neurologic deficits • Cervical involvement is less common than lumbar and thoracic involvement.

Fig. 5.3 a, b Unenhanced T2-weighted MR image (**a**) of spondylodiskitis at the C3/C4 level. The intervertebral disk is not delineated. Note the irregular contours of the vertebral body endplates and the hyperintense bone marrow in C3 and C4. Postgadolinium T1-weighted image (**b**) shows increased signal intensity of C3 and C4. The prevertebral space and spinal dural sac show inflammatory enhancement.

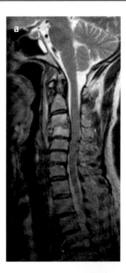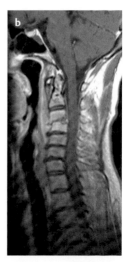

Fig. 5.4 Unenhanced T2-weighted MR image shows spondylodiskitis at C3/C4 with complete loss of the intervertebral disk space. The abscess wall is hypointense on the plain image and enhanced markedly after gadolinium administration (not shown).

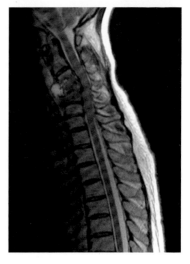

▶ **Treatment options**
Specific antibiotic therapy (usually *Staphylococcus aureus*) for several weeks ● Surgical intervention is limited to patients with neurological deficits, abscesses, vertebral body instability, or vertebral body deformity.

▶ **Course and prognosis**
Good prognosis ● Resolution takes up to 1 year, often culminates in spontaneous vertebral body fusion ● A neurologic deficit occurs in 25% of cases and is irreversible in 10% ● 5–10% mortality with antibiotic therapy, 14% incidence of reinfection ● Follow-up MRI is recommended to evaluate spinal integrity ● Enhancement after gadolinium administration may persist for several months even in the absence of acute infection.

Differential Diagnosis

Neoplastic process	– Often affects the entire vertebral body or posterior elements – Mass effect – Usually arises from the vertebral body – Convex posterior wall – Paired vertebral body involvement is uncommon
Epidural abscess	– Usually causes no signal changes in the vertebral body or disk
Rheumatoid spondylitis and other serum-negative spondylarthropathies	– Affect the atlantoaxial junction – Multifocal involvement is more common – Pannus formation, chronic (hypointense) destruction – Disk space narrowing; disk shows low or patchy signal intensity
Activated osteochondrosis	– Acute inflammatory exacerbation of significant osteochondrosis – Disk space may be narrowed but does not show increased signal intensity

Tips and Pitfalls

Failure to detect a secondary epidural abscess ● Activated osteochondrosis may be overinterpreted as spondylodiskitis.

Selected References

Barnes B, Alexander JT, Branch CL. Cervical osteomyelitis: a brief review. Neurosurg Focus 2004; 17(6)

Fernandez M, Carrol CL, Baker CJ. Discitis and vertebral osteomyelitis in children: an 18-year review. Pediatrics 2000; 105(6): 1299–1304

Lam KS, Webb JK. Discitis. Hosp Med 2004, 65(5): 280–286

Varma R, Lander P, Assaf A. Imaging of pyogenic infectious spondylodiskitis. Radiol Clin North Am 2001, 39: 203–213

Definition

▶ **Epidemiology**
Most common inflammation of the deep cervical soft tissues in children and adolescents • Usually develops from a tonsillar abscess • May spread to the para- and retropharyngeal tissues, masticator space, medial pterygoid muscle, and soft palate.

▶ **Etiology, pathophysiology, pathogenesis**
Usually self-limiting tonsillitis undergoes purulent liquefaction and spreads to the peritonsillar space • *Main causative organisms:* hemolytic group B streptococci, staphylococci, pneumococci, *Haemophilus* species.

Imaging Signs

▶ **Modality of choice**
CT, MRI.

▶ **CT findings**
Asymmetrical, inhomogeneous (peri)tonsillar mass • Contrast administration does not always produce typical ring enhancement • Frequent poor delineation of surrounding soft tissue structures • Frequently associated with cervical lymphadenitis.

▶ **MRI findings**
Increased T2-weighted signal intensity, increased T1-weighted signal intensity after gadolinium administration.

▶ **Pathognomonic findings**
Mass with an enhancing wall and small gas–fluid levels.

Clinical Aspects

▶ **Typical presentation**
Prior history of acute or chronic tonsillitis • Progressive neck pain and tonsillar swelling (edema) not controlled by oral antibiotics • Muffled "hot potato" voice • Persisting fever • Trismus in cases with pterygoid muscle involvement.

▶ **Treatment options**
Incision and drainage or needle aspiration • I.v. antibiotics (e.g., penicillin) • Tonsillectomy is usually delayed until inflammation subsides (after approximately 6 weeks) • "Hot" tonsillectomy is riskier but may be done to avoid a second operation.

▶ **Course and prognosis**
Excellent prognosis after surgical incision or needle aspiration and i.v. antibiotics • Reintervention may be necessary for further drainage • Withholding treatment may lead to abscess rupture and spontaneous drainage into the pharynx or surrounding fascial spaces.

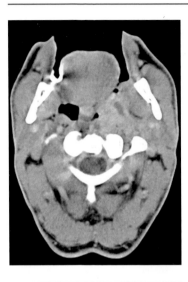

Fig. 5.5 Postcontrast CT of a left peritonsillar abscess. The mass has a hypodense center surrounded by an enhancing wall. Swelling of the left tonsil and ipsilateral pharyngeal mucosa has caused asymmetrical narrowing of the pharynx. The mouth is held open due to pain.

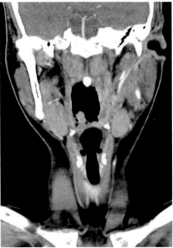

Fig. 5.6 Postcontrast CT (reformatted coronal image) of a left peritonsillar abscess shows perifocal swelling and increased enhancement of the mucosa. There is asymmetrical narrowing of the oropharynx extending caudally from the left side of the soft palate. The abscess shows typical peripheral enhancement with a central hypodense cavity.

Differential Diagnosis

Lymphoid hyperplasia	– Symmetrical, homogeneous enlargement of both tonsils – Enhancing intratonsillar septa
Tonsillar retention cyst	– Circumscribed tonsillar fluid collection – No perifocal edema – No enhancement after contrast administration
Dentogenic abscess	– Maxillary atrial involvement
Tonsillar involvement by non-Hodgkin lymphoma	– Unilateral submucous tumor mass – Nonenhancing septa – Pronounced, non-necrotizing lymphadenopathy
Tumors of the submucous salivary glands	– Benign: Sharply circumscribed, sometimes pedunculated growth – Malignant: Differentiation is required from carcinoma; lymphadenopathy is rare

Tips and Pitfalls

Avoid misinterpreting the tonsillar mass as a neoplasm.

Selected References

Mukherji SK, Castillo M. A simplified approach to the spaces of the extracranial head & neck. Radiol Clin North Am 1998; 36: 761–780

Schraff S. Peritonsillar abscess in children: A 10-year review of diagnosis and management. Int J Pediatr Otorhinlaryngol 2001; 57: 213–218

Windfuhr JP, Remmert S. Trends and complications in the management of peritonsillar abscess with emphasis on children. HNO 2004 Sep 24; E-pub [in press]

Definition

▶ **Epidemiology**
Accounts for 9% of all parapharyngeal masses ● Usually forms in the prestyloid compartment and spreads to the poststyloid compartment ● Streptococcal or staphylococcal infection is often present.

▶ **Etiology, pathophysiology, pathogenesis**
Purulent spread of inflammation within the parapharyngeal space ● Primary parapharyngeal infection is rare ● Usually invades the parapharyngeal space from adjacent structures ● Prestyloid cases arise from the tonsils and pharynx ● Rarely odontogenic ● May originate in the parotid gland or as an iatrogenic complication ● Poststyloid spread carries risk of cranial nerve lesions (CN IX–XII), jugular vein thrombosis, carotid aneurysm, and mediastinitis.

Imaging Signs

▶ **Modality of choice**
MRI, CT (87.9% sensitivity).

▶ **CT findings**
Increased parapharyngeal fat density that respects the cervical fasciae ● Inhomogeneous uni- or multilocular fluid or gas collection showing peripheral enhancement after contrast administration ● Perifocal edema.

▶ **MRI findings**
Diffuse increase in parapharyngeal signal intensity on T2-weighted images ● Abscess formation causes decreased T1-weighted signal intensity with perifocal enhancement after gadolinium administration (especially in fat-suppressed sequences) ● Liquefaction leads to high T2-weighted signal intensity ● Multiplanar views are necessary to evaluate extent.

▶ **Pathognomonic findings**
Inhomogeneous mass with an enhancing wall and small gas–fluid levels.

Clinical Aspects

▶ **Typical presentation**
When diagnosed, up to 50% of patients are already on antibiotics for ENT inflammatory disease ● Headache, neck pain and stiffness ● Drainage yields positive bacterial cultures in only about 50% of cases.

▶ **Treatment options**
Incision and drainage is an option only when an abscess is identified ● I. v. antibiotics (e.g., penicillin) may be appropriate in patients with pronounced cellulitis ● Without drainage, a mycotic aneurysm of the internal carotid artery may develop.

Fig. 5.7 Postcontrast CT of a right para-pharyngeal abscess shows an enhancing wall around a large, central hypodensity. Additional small abscesses can be seen lateral and anterior to the main abscess cavity. The parapharyngeal abscess has displaced the thyroid cartilage toward the left side.

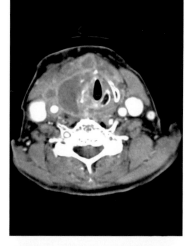

Fig. 5.8 Postcontrast CT of a retropha-ryngeal abscess shows a mass with low central density and a ring-enhancing wall located anterior to the cervical spine, just to the left of the midline. The submucous abscess has caused asymmetrical nar-rowing of the pharynx from the posterior left side.

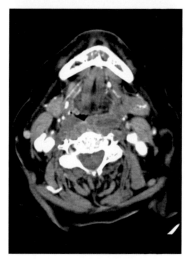

Differential Diagnosis

Parapharyngeal cellulitis	– Inhomogeneous enhancement of para-pharyngeal fat ("dirty fat") – Does not respect cervical fasciae
Primary cysts (branchial cleft cyst, dermoid, epidermoid)	– Frequently homogeneous, fluid-equivalent internal structure – Smooth, homogeneously enhancing walls
Benign tumor (e.g., cystic regressive adenoma)	– Inhomogeneous internal structure – Diffuse enhancement after contrast administration – Smooth margins – Low T1-weighted signal intensity, high T2-weighted signal intensity
Carcinoma	– Inhomogeneous internal structure – Diffuse enhancement after contrast administration – Indistinct margins that do not respect cervical fasciae
Cavitating lymph nodes	– Multiple lymph nodes – Normal-appearing fat – May have specific, e.g. tuberculous etiology
Thrombosis, aneurysm	– Vascular origin, usually homogeneous – High T1-weighted and T2-weighted signals

Tips and Pitfalls

It is difficult to distinguish between cellulitis and an abscess with MRI in children.

Selected References

Alaani A, Griffiths H, Minhas SS, Olliff J, Drake Lee AB. Parapharyngeal abscess: diagnosis, complications and management in adults. Eur Arch Otorhinolaryngol 2004

Sichel JY, Gomori JM, Sahh D, Elian J. Parapharyngeal abscess in children: the role of CT for diagnosis and treatment. Int J Pediatr Otorhinolaryngol 1996; 35: 213–222

Definition

▶ **Epidemiology**
Incidence of 10–35% ● Males are predominantly affected.
Nasopharynx: Increased incidence in Chinese (18%) ● 70–95% of all tumors of the nasopharynx, oropharynx, and hypopharynx.
Oropharynx and hypopharynx: Increased incidence in tobacco and alcohol misusers ● Frequency, spread, and lymph node involvement depend on the site of the lesion.

▶ **Etiology, pathophysiology, pathogenesis**
Most lesions are squamous cell carcinomas ● A smaller percentage are adenoid cystic carcinomas.
Nasopharynx: "Schmincke tumor" ● Associated with carcinogens and Epstein–Barr virus ● 90% incidence of lymph node involvement at diagnosis ● Three subtypes are distinguished:
- Type 1: Keratinizing.
- Type 2: Nonkeratinizing.
- Type 3: Undifferentiated.
Oropharynx: 80% tonsillar ● 15% soft palate ● 4% pharynx ● 60% incidence of lymph node involvement at diagnosis.
Hypopharynx: Frequent anaplastic ulcerating or exophytic growth ● 60% piriform sinus ● 25% retrocricoid ● 15% posterior pharyngeal wall ● 50% incidence of cervical lymph node involvement at diagnosis.

Imaging Signs

▶ **Modality of choice**
MRI, CT.

▶ **CT findings**
Invasive space-occupying lesion situated near the pharyngeal mucosa ● Often appears as an asymmetrical mass with irregular margins and moderate enhancement after contrast administration.

▶ **MRI findings**
Tumor is hypo- to isointense to muscle on T1-weighted images, clearly distinguishing it from fat ● Slightly hyperintense on T2-weighted images, where fat suppression aids in tumor delineation ● Minimal enhancement after gadolinium administration ● Better delineation in fat-suppressed sequences ● *Caution:* Tumor may infiltrate the neurovascular sheaths, bones, and muscles.

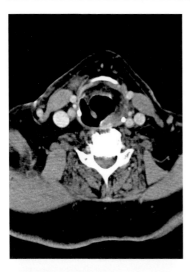

Fig. 5.9 Postcontrast CT of hypopharyngeal carcinoma shows a moderately enhancing tumor mass in the piriform recess, posterolateral to the mucosa, that has caused asymmetrical narrowing of the pharynx. The tumor has crossed the midline and invaded the parapharyngeal space on the left side.

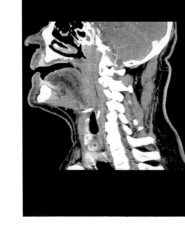

Fig. 5.10 Postcontrast CT of nasopharyngeal carcinoma (Schmincke tumor) reveals bony infiltration and local invasion of the skull base with intracranial tumor spread along the clivus. The tumor tissue has grown into the carotid canal (possible infiltration of the internal carotid artery). Note the lipomatous transformation of the lingual muscles resulting from tumor invasion of the ipsilateral hypoglossal nerve.

▶ **Pathognomonic findings**

Frequently inhomogeneous pharyngeal mass that may infiltrate adjacent structures, depending on the tumor stage.

AJCC staging of pharyngeal carcinoma:

- Nasopharynx: T1 (one subsite, submucous only) ● T2 (more than one subsite) ● T3 (nasal cavity, oropharynx) ● T4 (skull base, cranial nerves).
- Oropharynx: Tis (carcinoma in situ) ● T1 (< 2 cm) ● T2 (2–4 cm) ● T3 (> 4 cm) ● T4 (invasive growth).
- Hypopharynx: T1 (one subsite, ≤ 2 cm) ● T2 (more than one subsite or > 2 cm or < 4 cm without laryngeal fixation) ● T3 (> 4 cm or with laryngeal fixation) ● T4 (invasion of local structures).

Clinical Aspects

▶ **Typical presentation**

Often presents with nonspecific symptoms such as a painless, nonhealing mucosal ulcer ● Speech impairment ● Dysphagia ● Neurologic deficits only with T4 tumors ● Frequent lymph node involvement at diagnosis.

- *Nasopharyngeal metastasis* (decreasing frequency): Lymph nodes, bone, lung, liver.
- *Oropharyngeal metastasis* (decreasing frequency): Lymph nodes, lung, bone, liver.

▶ **Treatment options**

- *Nasopharynx:* Radiotherapy and brachytherapy.
- *Oropharynx:* Surgical excision ● Neck dissection plus radiochemotherapy.
- *Hypopharynx:* Radiochemotherapy ● Laryngopharyngectomy, depending on tumor stage.

▶ **Course and prognosis**

- *Nasopharynx:* Recurrences are common ● Endoscopy better for diagnosis.
- *Oropharynx:* 5-year survival rate with positive lymph nodes is less than 50%.
- *Hypopharynx:* Prognosis worsens in the following order: piriform sinus carcinoma, posterior wall carcinoma, retrocricoid carcinoma (5-year survival rate < 25%).

Differential Diagnosis

Tonsillar hyperplasia (naso- and oropharynx)	– Usually symmetrical, homogeneous enlargement of both tonsils – No invasive growth – Enhancing septa – Most patients < 20 years of age
Tonsillar involvement by non-Hodgkin lymphoma (naso- and oropharynx)	– Unilateral tumor mass spreading in the submucous plane – Pronounced, non-necrotizing lymph node enlargement
Benign salivary gland tumors (e.g., adenoma) (naso- and oropharynx)	– Noninvasive tumor with smooth margins – Tumor may be pedunculated and cause pharyngeal narrowing – No enhancing septa
Malignant salivary gland tumors (e.g., carcinoma) (naso-, oro- and hypopharynx)	– Adenoid cystic carcinoma, morphologically similar to squamous cell carcinoma – Often indistinguishable from squamous cell carcinoma – Lymph node metastases rare or absent
Kaposi sarcoma (hypopharynx)	– AIDS-associated neoplasia – Mucosal growth, similar to squamous cell carcinoma
Abscess	– Acute clinical symptoms – Abscess membrane

Tips and Pitfalls

A common error is to underestimate the degree of metastasis that has already occurred.

Selected References

Chin SC, Fatterpekar G, Chen CY, Som PM. MR imaging of diverse manifestations of nasopharyngeal carcinomas. AJR Am J Roentgenol 2003; 180(6): 1715–1722

Chung NN, Ting LL, Hsu WC, Lui LT, Wang PM. Impact of magnetic resonance imaging versus CT on nasopharyngeal carcinoma: primary tumor target delineation for radiotherapy. Head Neck 2004; 26(3): 241–246

Collaborative staging manual and coding instructions, version 1.0. Collaborative Staging Task Force of the American Joint Committee on Cancer 2004 NIH Publication Number 04–5496

Mukherji SK, Pillbury H, Castillo M. Imaging squamos cell carcinomas of the upper aerodigestive tract: what the clinicians need to know. Radiology 1997; 205: 629–646

Weber AL, Romo L, Hashmi S. Malignant tumors of the oral cavity and oropharynx: clinical, pathologic, and radiologic evaluation. Neuroimaging Clin N Am 2003; 13(3): 443–464

Definition

▶ **Epidemiology**

Males are predominantly affected by a 2:1 ratio • Peak incidence > 40 years of age • Congenital and acquired immune deficiency are predisposing • 10–20% of extranodal lymphomas occur in the head and neck, mostly in the Waldeyer ring • 50% of patients have lymph node involvement, 20% have gastrointestinal involvement.

▶ **Etiology, pathophysiology, pathogenesis**

NHL: Extranodal involvement of the palatine tonsil • *Malignant infiltration of MALT* (in decreasing frequency): Stomach, palatine tonsil (unilateral), nasopharyngeal adenoids (diffuse), lingual tonsil (unilateral) • Usually B-cell type • Slow local growth • Non-necrotizing.

Imaging Signs

▶ **Modality of choice**

MRI, CT.

▶ **CT findings**

Scan coverage extends from floor of sella turcica to infraclavicular level • Intense, homogeneous enhancement after contrast administration • Expansile mass not associated with destructive changes.

▶ **MRI findings**

Most tumors are unilateral • Expansile, nondestructive tonsillar mass • Enhances after gadolinium administration • No septa (DD: lymphoid hyperplasia with enhancing septa) • Increased, sometimes nonhomogeneous T2-weighted signal intensity.

▶ **Pathognomonic findings**

Cannot be positively distinguished from squamous cell carcinoma by imaging • NHL usually shows no bone destruction, even when extensive.

Clinical Aspects

▶ **Typical presentation**

Typical systemic manifestations (night sweats, fever, weight loss) may occur • Tumors at certain sites may cause dyspnea, dysphagia, and muffled nasal speech or other speech impediment • Otitis media • Neck and ear pain.

Clinical staging (Ann Arbor):

- Stage I: One lymph node region or one extranodal organ.
- Stage II: More than two lymph node regions or one extranodal region and more than one lymph node region on one side of the diaphragm.
- Stage III: Lymph node involvement on both sides of the diaphragm, with or without splenic or extranodal involvement.
- Stage IV: Diffuse or disseminated involvement of one or more extranodal organs, with or without lymph node involvement.

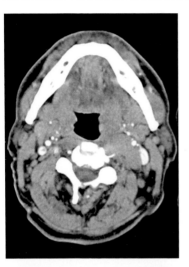

Fig. 5.11 Postcontrast CT of left tonsillar lymphoma shows diffuse, isodense swelling and infiltration of the lymphatic pharyngeal tissue at the maxillary level and slight, asymmetrical narrowing of the pharynx from the left side. The tumor has occluded the parapharyngeal fat spaces and displaced the left neurovascular sheath laterally.

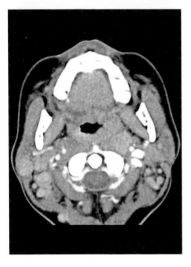

Fig. 5.12 Postcontrast CT shows circumferential lymphatic infiltration of the Waldeyer ring at the level of the palate in a patient with CLL. Multiple enlarged cervical lymph nodes show increased uptake of contrast medium.

▶ **Treatment options**

Combined radiotherapy and chemotherapy may be advised, depending on the tumor stage ● Stem cell transplantation may also be an option.

▶ **Course and prognosis**

Five-year survival rate ranges from 50% (stage I) to 10% (stage IV) ● Primary tonsillar NHL: No significant prognostic factor is known; radiochemotherapy is often curative.

Differential Diagnosis

Tonsillar hyperplasia (Waldeyer ring)	– Usually marked by symmetrical, homogeneous enlargement of both tonsils
	– Most patients under 20 years of age
	– No invasive growth
	– Enhancing intratonsillar septa
Squamous cell carcinoma (nasopharynx or oropharynx)	– Patients over 40 years of age
	– Tobacco and alcohol abuse
	– Painless ulcer
	– Possible necrotic lymph node metastases
Salivary gland tumors (nasopharynx or oropharynx)	– May be indistinguishable from lymphoma and squamous cell carcinoma
	– Lymph node metastases are rare

Tips and Pitfalls

It is difficult to distinguish tonsillar hyperplasia from tonsillar lymphoma.

Selected References

Cohnen M, Saleh A, Germing U, Engelbrecht V, Modder U. Imaging of supradiaphragmatic manifestations of extranodal non-Hodgkin's lymphoma. Radiologe 2002; 42(12): 960–969

Mohammadianpanah M, Omidvai S, Mosalei A, Ahmadloo N.Treatment results of tonsillar lymphoma: a 10-year experience. Ann Hematol 2005; 84(4): 223–226

Muller AM, Ihorst G, Mertelsmann R, Engelhardt M. Epidemiology of non-Hodgkin's lymphoma (NHL): trends, geographic distribution, and etiology. Ann Hematol 2004; 9

Anatomy

The larynx is divided into three anatomical levels:

- The supraglottic larynx, which is bounded superiorly by the ventricular folds, inferiorly by the vocal cords, anteriorly by the thyroid cartilage, and posteriorly and laterally by the aryepiglottic folds.
- The glottic larynx, consisting of the vocal cords, vocalis muscles, and laryngeal ventricles (sinus of Morgagni).
- The subglottic larynx, which extends below the vocal cords to the inferior border of the cricoid cartilage.

The aryepiglottic and thyroepiglottic muscles close the larynx during swallowing by their action on the epiglottis. An important barrier to supraglottic and subglottic tumor spread is the conus elasticus, a membrane between the cricoid and arytenoid cartilages that forms the free edge of the vocal cords. The inferior laryngeal nerve, the terminal branch of the recurrent laryngeal nerve, supplies all the laryngeal muscles except the cricopharyngeus, which is supplied by the superior laryngeal nerve. The posterior cricoarytenoid is the only muscle that abducts the vocal cords.

The primary pathway for lymphatic drainage of the larynx is along the internal jugular vein to the deep cervical lymph nodes and paratracheal lymph nodes.

The vocal cords appear hypointense on MRI. The ventricular folds appear hyperintense, particularly on T1-weighted images.

Definition

▶ **Epidemiology**

Laryngoceles are bilateral in 20–30% of cases • Internal laryngoceles are twice as common as external laryngoceles • Laryngoceles become infected in 8–10% of cases (infected laryngocele = laryngopyocele).

▶ **Etiology, pathophysiology, pathogenesis**

Rarely congenital, usually acquired • Dilatation of the sinus of Morgagni because of increased intraglottic pressure (straining, coughing, glass blowers, horn players) • *Rare causes:* Postinflammatory stenosis, tumor, trauma, tuberculosis • *Contents:* Air, fluid, pus.

– *Internal laryngoceles:* Protrude into the larynx, confined to the paraglottic space.

– *External (and mixed) laryngoceles:* Herniation through the thyrohyoid membrane between the superior border of the thyroid cartilage and the hyoid bone (saccular protrusions at a higher level are called pharyngoceles).

Imaging Signs

▶ **Modality of choice**

CT, MRI.

▶ **CT findings**

Sharply circumscribed mass with hypodense contents (isodense to air or fluid) and a thin wall • With external (mixed) laryngoceles, the internal component may collapse • Infected laryngoceles (laryngopyoceles) have a thickened, enhancing wall.

▶ **MRI findings**

Thin-walled cystic mass in the paraglottic space (internal) or extending into the soft tissues of the neck • Low T1-weighted signal intensity • T2-weighted signal intensity may be low (air) or high (fluid), depending on the contents • The origin of a laryngocele is best appreciated in coronal sequences.

▶ **Pathognomonic findings**

– *Internal laryngocele:* Air- or fluid-filled mass in the paraglottic space with protrusion of the vestibular fold.

– *External laryngocele:* Hourglass-shaped mass in the lower submandibular space • Air or fluid contents • Abuts against the thyrohyoid membrane • The narrow part of the hourglass corresponds to the site of membrane perforation.

Clinical Aspects

▶ **Typical presentation**

– *Internal laryngocele:* Hoarseness • Dyspnea • Stridor due to protrusion of the vestibular fold • Small ones are frequently asymptomatic.

– *External laryngocele:* Extends anteriorly into the neck below the mandibular angle • May have the same clinical manifestations as internal laryngocele,

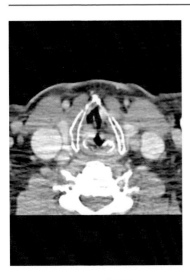

Fig. 6.1 Axial CT scan of an air-filled internal laryngocele on the right side.

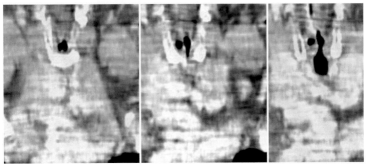

Fig. 6.2 Reformatted coronal images of the air-filled, thin-walled internal laryngocele in Fig. 6.**1**.

depending on the size of the internal component. Most common after 50 years of age ● Most prevalent in whites.

▶ **Treatment options**
 – *Internal laryngocele:* Endolaryngeal laser therapy.
 – *External laryngocele:* Excision through an external approach.

▶ **Course and prognosis**
 Gradual enlargement ● Good prognosis after treatment ● May recur.

▶ **What does the clinician want to know?**
 Familiarity with anatomic details prior to functional sinus surgery can prevent complications such as injuries to the anterior skull base, orbit, or optic nerve.

Differential Diagnosis

Thyroglossal cyst	– Develops from remnants of the thyroglossal duct
	– Cystic mass that abuts against the midportion of the hyoid bone
	– May be located in the center of the preepiglottic space
Hypopharyngeal diverticulum, Laimer diverticulum	– Fluid- or air-filled pseudodiverticulum of the lateral hypopharyngeal wall
Branchial cleft cyst	– No connection with the larynx
	– Can be palpated on the vascular sheath (anteromedial to the sternocleidomastoid muscle and lateral to the cervical vessels)

Tips and Pitfalls

A collapsed laryngocele is difficult to distinguish from a tumor • A secondarily infected laryngocele is difficult to distinguish from an abscess.

Selected References

Alvi A et al. Computed and magnetic resonance imaging characteristics of laryngocele and its variants. Am J Otolaryngol 1998; 19: 251–256

Canalis R et al. Laryngocele: an updated review. J Otolaryngol 1977; 6: 191–199

Glazer HS et al. Computed tomography of laryngoceles. AJR 1983; 140: 549–552

Koeller KK et al. Congenital cystic mass of the neck: Radiologic-Pathologic Correlation. Radiographics 1999; 19: 121–146

Thabet MH et al. Lateral saccular cysts of the larynx. Aetiology, diagnosis and management. J Laryngol Otol 2001; 115: 293–297

Definition

▶ **Epidemiology**
Most common in older white males • *Prevalence:* approximately 0.1–2% of all patients with dysphagia who have undergone diagnostic imaging.

▶ **Etiology, pathophysiology, pathogenesis**
Pseudodiverticulum • *Synonyms:* Pulsion diverticulum, hypopharyngeal diverticulum • Saccular protrusion of the hypopharyngeal mucosa at a weak point in the muscular posterior wall • *Location:* "Killian triangle" between the oblique and transverse fibers of the cricopharyngeus muscle (part of the inferior pharyngeal constrictor) • *Cause:* Motility disorder with altered compliance of the cricopharyngeal segment during the pharyngoesophageal phase of swallowing. *Associated esophageal changes:* Hiatal hernia (61%), gastroesophageal reflux (53%), abnormal peristalsis (46%), Barrett esophagus (15%).

Imaging Signs

▶ **Modality of choice**
Radiography (barium swallow).

▶ **Barium swallow**
Brombart classification:
- Stages I and II: Transient barium pool 2–10 mm wide above the cricopharyngeus posteromedial to the hypopharynx; empties spontaneously.
- Stage III: Barium pool more than 10 mm wide lasting minutes to hours • Crescent-shaped anteroinferior border formed by cricopharyngeus • No effect on the esophageal lumen.
- Stage IV: Barium pool more than 3 cm wide indenting and narrowing the cervical esophagus • Large diverticula usually extend posterolaterally toward the left side.

▶ **CT and MRI findings**
Usually an incidental finding • Air- or fluid-filled mass (may contain fluid levels) located behind and below the cricoid cartilage.

▶ **Other imaging modalities**
Ultrasonography • Oropharyngoesophageal scintigraphy (inflammation causes uptake of tracer in the diverticulum).

▶ **Pathognomonic findings**
Contrast pool posteroinferior to the cricoid cartilage that persists after oral administration of contrast • CT and MRI may demonstrate air or fluid contents and show direct contact of the mass with the hypopharynx.

Fig. 6.3 Zenker diverticulum impinging on the esophagus, demonstrated by barium swallow fluoroscopy. The PA projection (left) shows the diverticulum to the left of the midline. The lateral projection (right) shows the diverticulum as a barium-filled sac posterior to the esophagus.

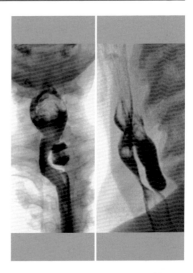

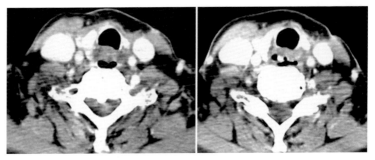

Fig. 6.4 CT demonstrates the diverticulum as an air-filled mass posterior to the collapsed esophagus.

Clinical Aspects

▶ **Typical presentation**
Dysphagia (does not correlate with size of diverticulum) ● Regurgitation ● Halitosis ● Aspiration ● Recurrent respiratory infections.

▶ **Treatment options**
Open surgical treatment via an external approach with excision and cricopharyngeal myotomy ● Diverticulopexy and myotomy ● Another option is endoscopic esophageal diverticulectomy.

▶ **Course and prognosis**
Gradual enlargement over a period of years ● May recur after surgery.
Complications (rare): Ulcer, perforation (caution: endoscopy, stomach tube), carcinoma, especially in large diverticula (incidence of 0.3–6.7%, usually with a long history of diverticulum, weight loss).

▶ **What does the clinician want to know?**
Diagnosis ● Extent of diverticulum ● Affected side ● Compression of adjacent structures.

Differential Diagnosis

Laimer diverticulum	– Lateral diverticulum below the cricopharyngeus (Laimer–Haeckerman triangle)
Cervical esophageal carcinoma	– Irregular boundaries – Infiltrating growth
Laryngocele	– Anterolateral to the esophagus in the paraglottic space

Tips and Pitfalls

Small Zenker diverticula are difficult to distinguish from cervical esophageal carcinoma on CT.

Selected References

Brombart M. Radiologie des Verdauungstraktes. Stuttgart: Thieme; 1973

Ekberg O. Neue chirurgisch-pathologische Aspekte des Zenker-Divertikels. Chirurg 1999; 70: 747–752

Kumoi K et al. Pharyngo-esophageal diverticulum arising from Laimer's triangle. Eur Arch Otorhinolaryngol 2001; 258: 184–187

Larynx

Definition

▶ **Epidemiology**
Common ● Hereditary angioedema is a somewhat rare cause (prevalence of approximately 2×10^{-6}).

▶ **Etiology, pathophysiology, pathogenesis**
Edematous swelling of the larynx and adjacent structures.
Causes: Trauma (intubation) ● Infection with viruses or Gram-negative bacteria (epiglottis) ● Allergic reaction (e.g., to contrast medium) ● Tumor (especially when infected) ● In up to 50% of cases, chronic laryngeal edema develops after radiotherapy for hypopharyngeal and glottic cancers. This is due to hyaline degeneration that leads to obstruction of laryngeal veins and lymphatics.
Special forms:
– Chronic hyperplastic laryngitis (Reinke edema): most common in smokers with vocal abuse.
– Acquired angioedema (caused by ACE inhibitors) or hereditary angioedema (caused by C1-esterase inhibitor deficiency, autosomal dominant, Quincke edema). *Precipitating factors:* Local trauma, hormonal changes, stress, certain foods and drugs.
– Laryngopharyngeal reflux disease: caused by gastroesophageal reflux.

Imaging Signs

▶ **Modality of choice**
CT.

▶ **CT findings**
Usually shows hypodense thickening of the affected portions of the larynx ● Usually symmetrical when caused by allergy, angioedema, infectious laryngitis, or radiotherapy ● Often asymmetrical when caused by a tumor ● Reinke edema marked by unilateral or bilateral polypoid thickening of the vocal cords ● Mucosal enhancement is seen mainly with inflammation and tumors ● Chronic laryngeal edema after radiotherapy often shows increased density of the paralaryngeal, paraglottic, and subcutaneous fat plus thickening of the platysma and skin (difficult to distinguish from local recurrence).

▶ **MRI findings**
Thickening of the affected laryngeal mucosa ● Low T1-weighted signal intensity, high T2-weighted signal intensity ● Postgadolinium enhancement when edema is due to inflammation or tumor ● Radiation-induced chronic laryngeal edema shows decreased T1-weighted signal intensity in the paralaryngeal space.

▶ **Pathognomonic findings**
– *Reinke edema:* Unilateral or bilateral thickening of the vocal cords.
– *Quincke edema:* Diffuse laryngeal edema; may also affect the epiglottis, subglottis, or esophagus.
– *Laryngopharyngeal reflux disease:* Supraglottic, glottic, and subglottic edema, pronounced thickening of the mucosa in the posterior commissure (arytenoid cartilage area).

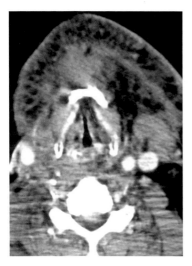

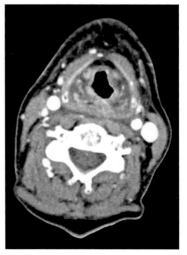

Fig. 6.5 CT in a man who underwent radiotherapy and right-sided neck dissection for carcinoma of the tongue. The scan shows inhomogeneous increased density and swelling of the laryngeal soft tissue and subcutaneous fat as a sign of radiation-induced edema.

Fig. 6.6 CT scan of a woman with laryngeal edema shows circumferential, hypodense mucosal swelling.

- *Chronic laryngeal edema after radiotherapy:* Thickening of the epiglottis, aryepiglottic fold, ventricular fold, posterior pharyngeal wall, anterior and posterior glottic commissures, and subglottic mucosa. Edema of the retropharyngeal space.

Clinical Aspects

▶ **Typical presentation**
With hereditary angioedema, edema is often found in the limbs, bowel (acute abdomen), and urogenital tract (micturition difficulties) ● Peak occurrence: 10–30 and after 50 years of age ● Edema associated with an infectious or allergic etiology or angioedema generally presents with acute symptoms ● Tumor-associated and postirradiation edema presents with chronic symptoms. Acute and chronic symptoms include inspiratory stridor, harsh voice, hoarseness, cough, dysphagia, foreign body sensation, and/or dyspnea ● Infections present with fever.

▶ **Treatment options**
- *Infection:* Antibiotics ● Corticosteroids.
- *Allergy:* Corticosteroids ● Antihistamines ● Volume infusion.

- *Acquired angioedema:* Withdraw the antigen (ACE inhibitor) • Corticosteroids • Antihistamines.
- *Hereditary angioedema:* C1 INH replacement • Tranexamic acid • Interval therapy with danazol • Corticosteroids • Antihistamines • Epinephrine is ineffective!
- *Acute dyspnea*: Intubation or tracheotomy.
- *Reinke edema:* Decortication of the vocal cords.
- *Laryngopharyngeal reflux:* Treatment of underlying disease (proton pump inhibitor, upper body elevation, fundoplication).

▶ **Course and prognosis**

Angioedema and allergic forms show rapid clinical improvement with treatment • In patients with hereditary angioedema, there is a 12% mortality rate from suffocation due to glottic edema • Infectious forms and gastroesophageal reflux tend to have a favorable course • Chronic laryngeal edema after radiotherapy is very resistant to treatment • Asymmetry should raise suspicion of local recurrence.

▶ **What does the clinician want to know?**

Extent of edema • Changes in surrounding structures • Asymmetry – which may indicate a tumor or local recurrence (e.g., after radiotherapy).

Differential Diagnosis

Glottic carcinoma, supraglottic carcinoma	– Difficult to distinguish from chronic laryngeal edema after radiotherapy
	– Most important criterion: asymmetry of mucosal thickening plus infiltration or destruction of adjacent structures
Paralaryngeal abscess	– Complication of laryngitis or trauma
	– Liquid center
	– Enhancing wall
Wegener granulomatosis	– Most commonly affects the paranasal sinuses
	– Possible concomitant involvement of hypopharynx and larynx
	– Inflammatory edema, often accompanied by cartilage destruction

Tips and Pitfalls

Asymmetry, though nonspecific, is often the only criterion for distinguishing tumor from edema • Always consider the possibility of bilateral glottic carcinoma.

Selected References

Dietz A et al. Das chronische Larynxödem als Spätreaktion nach Radiochemotherapie. HNO 1998; 46: 731–738

Göring HD et al. Untersuchung zum hereditären Angioödem im deutschsprachigen Raum. Hautarzt 1998; 49: 114–122

Mukherji SK et al. Radiologic appearance of the irradiated larynx. Part I. Expected changes. Radiology 1994; 193(1): 141–148

Definition

▶ **Epidemiology**
Most important traumatic injury of the larynx and hypopharynx.

▶ **Etiology, pathophysiology, pathogenesis**
Blunt trauma (e.g., motor vehicle injury, fist fight, strangulation, fall) ● Frequent associated hematoma, bleeding, and edema of the laryngeal soft tissues ● Mucosal laceration may lead to soft-tissue emphysema.

Imaging Signs

▶ **Modality of choice**
CT.

▶ **CT findings**
Fracture line (usually anterior) ● Paralaryngeal hematoma (fresh bleeding is hyperintense), may cause tracheal displacement ● Rarely, there is extravasation of contrast because of persistent bleeding ● Subcutaneous air collection is usually seen with soft-tissue emphysema.
Possible dislocation of the arytenoid cartilage: Unphysiologic position or rotation of the arytenoid cartilage ● Swelling of the aryepiglottic fold ● Vocal cord fixation during "E" phonation or Valsalva maneuver.

▶ **MRI findings**
MRI may demonstrate a fracture line ● Hematoma may be hyper-, iso- or hypointense to muscle on T1- and T2-weighted images, depending on the age of the collection ● No enhancement after gadolinium administration.

▶ **Pathognomonic findings**
CT shows discontinuity in the thyroid cartilage (fracture line) ● Accompanying hematoma ● Broadening of the laryngeal and paratracheal soft-tissue shadow on conventional radiographs (lateral projection of cervical spine).

Clinical Aspects

▶ **Typical presentation**
Subcutaneous hematoma at the level of the larynx ● Acute dyspnea ● Dysphagia ● Stridor ● Hemoptysis ● Dysphonia ● Odynophagia.

▶ **Treatment options**
– *Undisplaced fracture:* Antibiotics ● Corticosteroids ● I.v. calcium ● Ice collar.
– *Displaced fracture:* Open reduction ● Fracture of the laryngeal skeleton requires tracheotomy and internal splinting of the larynx with a plastic stent.

▶ **Course and prognosis**
Usually favorable course with early treatment ● Risk of chronic laryngeal or tracheal stenosis with poor initial treatment ● Postoperative dysphonia is common after a severely displaced fracture.

▶ **What does the clinician want to know?**
Precise location ● Displacement ● Complications.

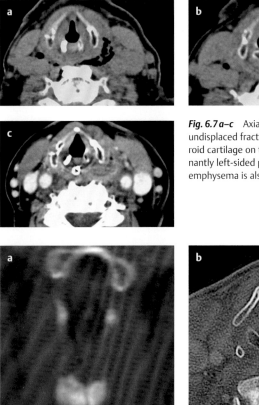

Fig. 6.7 a–c Axial CT scans of a traumatic, undisplaced fracture of the posterior thyroid cartilage on the right side. Predominantly left-sided paralaryngeal soft-tissue emphysema is also seen.

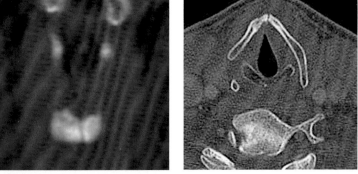

Fig. 6.8 a, b Coronal and axial CT images of an old fracture of the anterior commissure of the thyroid cartilage.

Differential Diagnosis

Tumor infiltration (stage T4)	– CT: cortical discontinuity, moderate enhancement – MRI: high T2-weighted signal intensity, indistinct margins
Ossification	– CT: negative central attenuation values (fat marrow) – MRI: high T1-weighted signal intensity

Tips and Pitfalls

An adequate FOV is necessary to evaluate head or neck injuries with an uncertain trauma mechanism ● Consider the possibility of laryngeal injury even in the absence of obvious laryngeal bruising.

Selected References

Bent JP, Porubsky ES. The management of blunt fractures of the thyroid cartilage. Otolaryngol. Head Neck Surg 1994; 110: 195–202

Ganzel TM, Mumford LA. Diagnosis and management of acute laryngeal trauma. Am Surg 1989; 55(5): 303–306

Schaefer SD, Brown OE. Selective application of CT in the management of laryngeal trauma. Laryngoscope 1983; 93: 1473–1475

Schild JA, Denneny EC. Evaluation and treatment of acute laryngeal fractures. Head Neck 1989; 11(6): 491–496

Definition

▶ **Epidemiology**
Rare • More common at thoracic or lumbar level.

▶ **Etiology, pathophysiology, pathogenesis**
Usually results from hematogenous spread • Rare complication of anterior or posterior instrumentation of the cervical spine (in 0.5% of operations) • Trauma or perforation of the hypopharynx or cervical esophagus (direct shearing forces from bone fragments or spondylophytes; injury during surgical intervention) • Complication of epidural abscess or cervical spondylodiskitis • *Causative organisms: Staphylococcus aureus*, less commonly *Streptococcus pyogenes* or *Mycobacterium tuberculosis* • *Predisposing factors:* Weakened host defenses (e.g., diabetes mellitus, HIV, i.v. drug abuse).

Imaging Signs

▶ **Modality of choice**
CT.

▶ **CT findings**
Prevertebral mass • Central low attenuation • Possible gas inclusions • Increased density of adjacent fatty tissue • Peripheral rim enhancement after contrast administration • Bone erosion due to precipitating or accompanying spondylitis or diskitis.

▶ **MRI findings**
High central T2-weighted signal intensity, low T1-weighted signal intensity • Enhancement of surrounding membrane after gadolinium administration • Increased T2-weighted signal intensity of surrounding tissue due to perifocal inflammatory reaction • Possible susceptibility artifacts caused by gas inclusions.

▶ **Radiographic findings**
Lateral projection: Broadening of the prevertebral space • Possible prevertebral gas inclusion • Erosion of adjacent vertebral bodies due to concomitant spondylitis or diskitis.

▶ **Pathognomonic findings**
Prevertebral liquid mass with relatively well-defined margins and an enhancing membrane • Possible gas inclusions and perifocal inflammatory reaction • Possible signs of spondylodiskitis.

Clinical Aspects

▶ **Typical presentation**
Signs of infection (fever, leukocytosis, raised CRP) • Pain exacerbated by head turning and flexion/extension of the cervical spine • Dysphagia • Stiff neck • Causal or concomitant epidural abscess may lead to meningism, root symptoms, or muscle weakness in all four limbs.

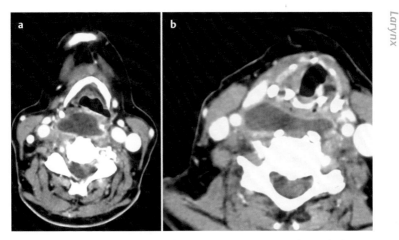

Fig. 6.9 a, b　Large prevertebral abscess at the level of the larynx, displacing the larynx anteriorly and to the left. Scan (**a**) also shows a mediolateral epidural abscess on the left side.

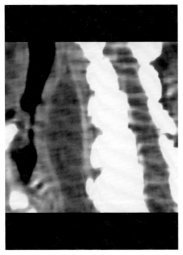

Fig. 6.10　Reformatted sagittal image defines the craniocaudal extent of the abscess.

▶ **Treatment options**

I.v. antibiotics ● Drainage of abscess ● Eradication of inflammatory foci (e.g., internal fixation material) ● *Epidural abscess:* Laminectomy and drainage ● *Hypopharyngeal or esophageal perforation or fistula:* Surgical treatment.

▶ **Course and prognosis**

Prompt diagnosis and treatment should lead to a favorable course and full recovery ● *Possible complications:* Scar contractions of the hypopharynx or cervical esophagus ● Fistulation to the pharynx, esophagus, or spine ● Epidural abscess ● Spondylodiskitis ● Neurologic deficits ● Delayed treatment may lead to fatal outcome.

▶ **What does the clinician want to know?**

Diagnosis ● Level of the abscess ● Extent ● Complications.

Differential Diagnosis

Zenker diverticulum	– Air- or fluid-filled mass posteroinferior to the cricoid cartilage
	– May contain air–fluid level
	– Perifocal reaction is rare
Cervical chordoma	– Rare
	– Erosion or destruction of adjacent vertebral body, internal septation, amorphous calcifications
	– Moderate enhancement after contrast administration
Esophageal carcinoma	– Irregular prevertebral mass
	– May show central necrosis
	– May not be delineated from the esophagus
	– Intraluminal tumor component

Tips and Pitfalls

Carefully evaluate the epidural space, vertebral bodies, and intervertebral disks at the level of the lesion to detect possible complications or determine the cause ● Consider a mycobacterial etiology in immunosuppressed patients.

Selected References

Davis W et al. CT and MRI of the normal and diseased perivertebral space. Neuroradiology 1995; 37: 388–394

Kim YJ, Glazer PA. Delayed esophageal perforation and abscess formation after cervical vertebrectomy and fusion. Orthopedics 2002; 25: 1091–1093

Talmi YP et al. Postsurgical prevertebral abscess of the cervical spine. Laryngoscope 2000; 110 (7): 1137–1141

Definition

▶ **Epidemiology**
Accounts for 2.5% of all cancers in men and 0.5% in women ● 50% of all head and neck cancers ● 30% of all laryngeal carcinomas are supraglottic ● 40% of tumors have already metastasized to deep lateral cervical lymph nodes when diagnosed.

▶ **Etiology, pathophysiology, pathogenesis**
Carcinoma of the superficial epithelium of the epilarynx (suprahyoid epiglottis to arytenoid area) or supraglottis (infrahyoid epiglottis to ventricular folds) ● Most tumors are keratinizing or nonkeratinizing squamous cell carcinomas ● *Cause:* exogenous toxins (e.g., nicotine, alcohol) ● *Possible preexisting diseases:* chronic laryngitis, pachydermia, leukoplakia, papillomas.
Classification:
– T1: Limited to one subsite with normal vocal cord mobility.
– T2: Invades the mucosa of more than one adjacent subsite of the supraglottis or an area outside the supraglottis (e.g., vallecula or piriform sinus) with normal vocal fold mobility.
– T3: Limited to the larynx with vocal fold fixation and/or invades the postcricoid area, preepiglottic tissue, or paraglottic space, with slight erosion of the thyroid cartilage.
– T4a: Extends through the thyroid cartilage to the soft tissues of the neck, extrinsic lingual muscles, neck strap muscles, thyroid gland, and esophagus.
– T4b: Extends into the prevertebral space, mediastinal structures, internal carotid artery.

Imaging Signs

▶ **Modality of choice**
Contrast-enhanced CT

▶ **CT findings**
Fast spiral CT is the staging method of choice due to potential motion artifacts (coughing, swallowing) ● Asymmetry of supraglottic luminal boundaries ● Significant enhancement after contrast administration ● Infiltrating, invasive growth ● Cartilage and bone destruction.

▶ **MRI findings**
Asymmetrical mass with low to intermediate T1-weighted signal intensity and high T2-weighted signal intensity ● Increased signal intensity in PD-weighted sequences ● Significant (homogeneous or inhomogeneous) enhancement after gadolinium administration ● Infiltrating, invasive growth ● MRI is excellent for evaluating cartilage infiltration.

▶ **PET, PET-CT**
PET can stage lymph node involvement and detect recurrence with high sensitivity and specificity ● Good spatial resolution of lesions with increased cellular metabolism.

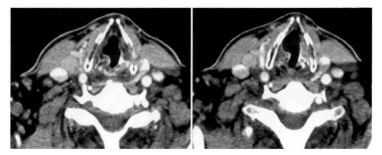

Fig. 6.11 Contrast-enhanced CT scans of a right-sided supraglottic carcinoma. The tumor has not transgressed the midline. It shows only slight enhancement, and the mass effect on the laryngeal lumen is the main CT finding.

▶ **Pathognomonic findings**
Enhancing mass • Infiltration of deep layers of the larynx including preepiglottic tissue and paraglottic space • Large tumors are associated with destruction of thyroid cartilage • Lymph node metastases.
Criteria for a malignant tumor: Asymmetrical, infiltrating growth • Ill-defined margins • Inhomogeneous internal structure.

Clinical Aspects

▶ **Typical presentation**
Occurs predominantly in older men • Feeling of pressure in the larynx • Foreign body sensation • Swallowing difficulties • Later, harsh voice and hoarseness • Aspiration • Many tumors are clinically silent for some time and are not diagnosed until lymph node enlargement is noted.

▶ **Treatment options**
T1 and T2 tumors can be removed by endolaryngeal laser surgery • Tumors involving the epiglottis and vestibular fold but sparing the vocal cords can be removed by a horizontal supraglottic partial laryngectomy • Larger tumors require a total laryngectomy • Metastases require neck dissection and postoperative radiotherapy.

▶ **Course and prognosis**
Five-year survival rate is approximately 60–75% • Tumors near the glottis have a better prognosis because they become symptomatic at an earlier stage.

▶ **What does the clinician want to know?**
Extent of disease • Changes in adjacent structures • Spread across the midline • Metastases.

Differential Diagnosis

Chondrosarcoma	– Originates from the thyroid or cricoid cartilage
	– Amorphous calcified matrix

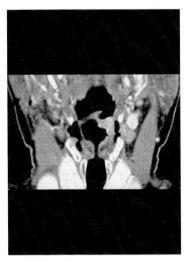

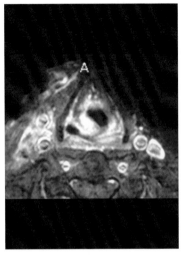

Fig. 6.12 MPR of cervical CT in another patient shows an enhancing mass in the supraglottic space.

Fig. 6.13 A right-sided carcinoma appears hyperintense on a fat-suppressed T1-weighted image after gadolinium administration.

Arytenoid arthritis	– History of rheumatoid arthritis – Localized edema with decreased motion of the arytenoid cartilage
Rhabdomyosarcoma, fibrosarcoma, adenoid cystic sarcoma	– Indistinguishable from squamous cell carcinoma – May show atypical location; direction of growth along muscular structures and tendon insertions

Tips and Pitfalls

Endoscopic examination is helpful in increasing the accuracy of radiologic staging •
Spread across the midline may not be detected by imaging.

Selected References

Castelijns JA et al. Imaging of laryngeal cancer. Semin Ultrasound CT MR 1998; 19: 492–504

Steinkamp HJ et al. Wertigkeit von Magnetresonanztomographie und Computertomographie im Tumorstaging des Larynx-/Hypopharynxkarzinoms. Fortschr Röntgenstr 1993; 158: 437–444

Vogl TJ et al. MRI with Gd-DTPA in Tumors of Larynx and Hypopharynx. Eur Radiol 1991; 1: 58–64

Definition

▶ **Epidemiology**

Incidence: 0.5 % of all carcinomas ● 95 % are squamous cell carcinomas ● 60 % of all laryngeal carcinomas are glottic ● 10 % incidence of lymph node involvement on initial diagnosis (vocal cords are avascular and also do not have lymphatics).

▶ **Etiology, pathophysiology, pathogenesis**

Carcinoma of the vocal cords, anterior or posterior commissure ● Keratinizing to moderately differentiated squamous cell carcinoma ● *Cause:* Exogenous toxins (nicotine, alcohol) ● *Possible preexisting conditions:* Chronic laryngitis, pachydermia, leukoplakia, papillomas.

Classification:

– T1: Limited to vocal cord(s) with normal vocal cord mobility.
– T2: Extension to supraglottis or subglottis with impaired vocal cord mobility.
– T3: Vocal fold fixation, extension to preepiglottic space, slight erosion of the thyroid cartilage.
– T4a: Extends through the thyroid cartilage to the soft tissues of the neck, extrinsic lingual muscles, neck strap muscles, thyroid gland, and esophagus.
– T4b: Extends into the prevertebral space, mediastinal structures, internal carotid artery.

Imaging Signs

▶ **Modality of choice**

Contrast-enhanced CT.

▶ **CT findings**

Fast spiral CT is the staging method of choice due to possible motion artifacts (coughing, swallowing) ● Enhancing soft-tissue mass of the vocal cord(s) ● Infiltrating or exophytic growth.

▶ **MRI findings**

Mass with low to intermediate T1-weighted signal intensity and high T2-weighted signal intensity ● Homogeneous enhancement after gadolinium administration ● MRI is excellent for evaluating cartilage infiltration.

▶ **Pathognomonic findings**

Moderately enhancing, invasive, or exophytic mass arising from the vocal cord ● *Patterns of spread:* Anteromedial to anterior commissure, posterior to arytenoid or cricoid cartilage, subglottic extension, or supraglottic extension into the paraglottic space.

Clinical Aspects

▶ **Typical presentation**

Occurs predominantly in older men ● Hoarseness ● Voice change ● Later, respiratory distress ● Any hoarseness that persists for 3–4 weeks is suspicious for carcinoma ● *Endoscopic finding:* Unilateral redness of affected vocal cord, which is thickened, nodulated, ulcerated, and coated with fibrin.

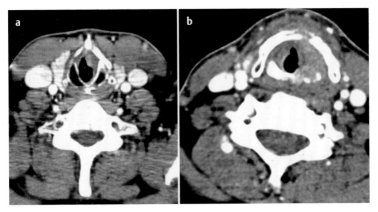

Fig. 6.14 a, b Left-sided enhancing laryngeal carcinoma without cartilaginous invasion (**a**). Extensive laryngeal carcinoma with destruction of the left arytenoid cartilage and the posterosuperior portion of the cricoid cartilage (**b**).

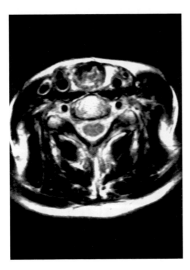

Fig. 6.15 The subglottic part of the carcinoma appears inhomogeneously isointense to hyperintense on the T2-weighted MR image, which documents spread across the midline.

▶ **Treatment options**

T1 tumors can be treated by endolaryngeal laser resection or percutaneous radiotherapy (60 Gy) • Larger tumors require a combination of radiotherapy and partial or total laryngectomy • Invasion of the anterior commissure requires a vertical Leroux–Robert frontolateral resection.

▶ **Course and prognosis**

Relatively favorable prognosis owing to late metastasis and early clinical manifestations • Five-year survival rate of T1 tumors is approximately 95% after operative treatment or radiotherapy • Five-year survival rate of T4 tumors is approximately 25%.

Differential Diagnosis

Rheumatoid arthritis of arytenoid joint	– History of rheumatoid arthritis – Local edema with decreased mobility of the arytenoid cartilage
Chondrosarcoma	– Arises from the cricoid or thyroid cartilage – Amorphous calcified matrix
Wegener granulomatosis of the larynx	– Glottic and supraglottic thickening – Concomitant renal, nasal, or pulmonary involvement
Papilloma	– Same clinical manifestations (hoarseness) as glottic carcinoma – Smooth margins with cauliflower-like morphology of the anterior aspect of the vestibular fold or vocal cord

Tips and Pitfalls

Endoscopic examination is very helpful for increasing the accuracy of radiologic staging • Differentiation between recurrent or residual tumor and postactinic changes (edema) may be difficult following radiotherapy.

Selected References

Castelijns JA et al. Imaging of laryngeal cancer. Semin Ultrasound CT MR 1998; 19: 492–504

Steinkamp HJ et al. Wertigkeit von Magnetresonanztomographie und Computertomographie im Tumorstaging des Larynx-/Hypopharynxkarzinoms. Fortschr Röntgenstr 1993; 158: 437–444

Vogl TJ et al. MRI with Gd-DTPA in Tumors of Larynx and Hypopharynx. Eur Radiol 1991; 1: 58–64

Definition

Cavitary lesion (fissural cyst, pseudocyst, or soft-tissue cyst) of the maxilla or mandible not originating from the tooth or its derivatives • Uni- or multilocular • Fluid-containing or semisolid • May have epithelial lining.

▶ **Epidemiology**

Can occur at any age • Males predominantly affected • Maxilla affected more often than mandible • Frequently an incidental finding.

▶ **Etiology, pathophysiology, pathogenesis**

Epithelial remnants of the nasopalatine canal (incisive canal cyst) or the union of the embryonic globular and maxillary processes (globulomaxillary cyst) • Etiology of aneurysmal and solitary bone cysts is uncertain.

▶ **Clinical classification:**

- *Lined with epithelium:* Nasopalatine = median fissural (incisive canal) cyst, lateral fissural (globulomaxillary) cyst, nasal vestibular cyst.
- *Not lined with epithelium* (pseudocyst): Stafne cyst, aneurysmal and solitary (traumatic, hemorrhagic) bone cysts.
- *Soft-tissue cysts:* Retention cyst, gingival cyst, dermoid cyst.

Imaging Signs

▶ **Modality of choice**

MRI, CT.

▶ **CT findings**

Well-circumscribed cystic lesion in the maxilla or mandible • May contain fluid • Does not enhance after contrast administration • Some aneurysmal bone cysts are multilocular • Blood-filled lumen creates a fluid level.

▶ **MRI findings**

Well-circumscribed mass • May show inhomogeneous T1- and T2-weighted signal intensity, depending on protein content • Does not enhance after gadolinium administration • Aneurysmal bone cyst: Fluid–fluid level due to intralesional hemorrhage • Caution: Define precise relationship to neurovascular bundle, periodontium, and dental pulp.

▶ **Pathognomonic findings**

Location and appearance of a benign bone cyst • Fluid–fluid level in aneurysmal bone cyst • Even with a typical presentation, histologic confirmation is advised.

Clinical Aspects

▶ **Typical presentation**

Usually an incidental finding • Intraoral or extraoral swelling • Pain or inflammation • Loosening of teeth • Tooth displacement • Tooth loss • Pathologic fracture.

Aneurysmal bone cyst: Grows rapidly • Causes bone expansion (proliferative rather than expansile growth).

Fig. 7.1 Solitary nonodontogenic bone cyst in the left molar region of the maxilla. Plain CT with bone window setting shows a well-circumscribed mass with displacement and thinning of the cortex. Note the sclerotic wall and soft-tissue density of the contents. The mass is not in contact with any teeth.

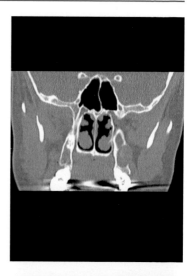

Fig. 7.2 Globulomaxillary (lateral fissural) cyst. Incidental finding on plain T2-weighted MR image in a patient with squamous cell carcinoma of the left maxillary sinus located laterally in the maxilla, affecting the region of the incisors and canines. The teeth are displaced, and the cyst does not contain any dental tissues.

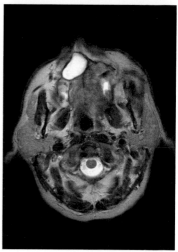

▶ **Treatment options**
Cystectomy or cystotomy ● Extraction or apical root resection of affected teeth may be required.
▶ **Course and prognosis**
Surgical treatment is curative ● Incidental findings usually do not require follow-up.

Differential Diagnosis

Odontogenic cyst: radicular, follicular or keratocyst	– Often related to a tooth or an empty alveolus – Usually have an inflammatory cause with corresponding clinical features – Radicular cyst causes widening of the periodontal space
Benign neoplasms: ameloblastoma, odontogenic tumors, fibroma, myxoma	– Extracystic tissue can often be identified – Greater expansile growth and mass effect – Usually show more intense contrast enhancement
Malignant neoplasms: sarcoma, myeloma, secondary invasion by carcinoma	– Often there are signs of extracystic tissue infiltration – May develop in the wall of follicular cysts – Greater vestibulolingual extent

Tips and Pitfalls

Nasopalatine cysts are usually very small and are often missed.

Selected References

Kress G, Gottschalk A, Schmitter M, Sartor K. Benigne Erkrankungen des Unterkiefers im MRT. Fortschr Röntgenstr 2004; 176(4): 491–499

Weber A, Kaneda T, Scrivani S, Aziz S. Jaw: cysts, tumors, and nontumorous lesions. In: Som P, Curtin H, eds. Head and neck imaging. St. Louis: Mosby; 2003: 319–349

Yoshiura K, Weber AL, Runnels S, Scrivani SJ. Cystic lesions of the mandible and maxilla. Neuroimaging Clin N Am 2003; 13(3): 485–494

Definition

▶ **Epidemiology**

Most common congenital malformation of the neck ● 65% infrahyoid, 15% suprasternal ● Common in children < 10 years ● 10–65% of patients are < 35 years of age ● No sex predilection ● Sinus tract or fistula usually a result of rupture or incision of an infected cyst.

▶ **Etiology, pathophysiology, pathogenesis**

Neck cyst arising from the thyroglossal duct and located on or near the midline ● Failure of involution of the thyroglossal duct (week 6 of embryonic development) ● Persistence of secretory epithelium leads to cyst development ● May become infected ● Ectopic thyroid tissue may occur (10–45% of cases).

Imaging Signs

▶ **Modality of choice**

MRI, CT.

▶ **CT findings**

Rounded, hypodense, nonenhancing mass ● *Site of occurrence:* Foramen cecum of the tongue; extends through or past the hyoid bone, in front of the cricoid and infrahyoid muscles as far as the thyroid gland ● An ectopic thyroid is marked by intensely enhancing tissue.

▶ **MRI findings**

Benign cystic mass, usually round in shape ● Thin enhancing wall ● Low T1-weighted signal intensity, high T2-weighted signal intensity.

▶ **Pathognomonic findings**

Median cyst ● Bland cyst embedded in the infrahyoid muscles ● The more caudal the level of the cyst, the further it is from the midline.

Clinical Aspects

▶ **Typical presentation**

Recurrent, usually asymptomatic anterior neck mass ● Situated in or near the midline ● Soft consistency ● Moves with swallowing ● Superinfection leads to pain and dysphagia.

▶ **Treatment options**

Cystectomy or cystotomy ● Recurrence is minimized by also removing the midportion of the hyoid bone and its extension to the foramen cecum.

▶ **Course and prognosis**

Excellent cure rates (5% recurrence rate) ● Secondary infection is rare.

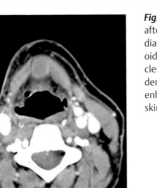

Fig. 7.3 Thyroglossal duct cyst. CT scan after contrast administration. The median cyst is located just caudal to the hyoid bone between the thyrohyoid muscles. The cyst contents are slightly hypodense to muscle and surrounded by a thin enhancing wall. The cyst did not reach skin level and was an incidental finding.

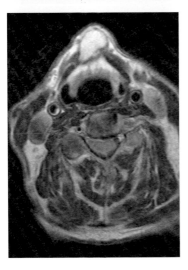

Fig. 7.4 Thyroglossal duct cyst. Plain T2-weighted MR image shows a well-circumscribed cyst just caudal to the hyoid bone with hyperintense contents and a hypointense wall. The cyst formed a clinically visible bulge in the skin.

Differential Diagnosis

Lymph node enlargement (inflammatory, malignant)	– Central contrast enhancement (in the absence of central necrosis) – Difficult to distinguish from infected thyroglossal duct cyst—note location!
Thyroid adenoma of the isthmus or pyramidal lobe	– Usually forms a solid, enhancing mass – Hyperintense to thyroglossal duct cyst on T1-weighted images
Dermoid	– Located in the tongue, for example – May contain hair follicles or hair – High T1-weighted signal intensity, isodense with fat on CT (fat content)
Abscess	– Inflammatory reaction in surrounding tissue – Enhancing wall
Hematoma	– No enhancing wall – Typical CT density, inhomogeneous signal intensity on MRI
External laryngocele	– Usually has demonstrable relationship to the larynx – Usually has a more lateral location; contains air or fluid

Tips and Pitfalls

Avoid diagnostic confusion with abscess and hematoma.

Selected References

Brousseau VJ, Solares CA, Xu M, Krakovitz P, Koltai PJ. Thyroglossal duct cysts: presentation and management in children versus adults. Int J Pediatr Otorhinolaryngol 2003; 67(12): 1285–1290

Mahboubi S, Gheyi V. MR imaging of airway obstruction in infants and children. Int J Pediatr Otorhinolaryngol 2001; 57(3): 219–227

Tas A, Karasalihoglu AR, Yagiz R, Doganay L, Guven S. Thyroglossal duct cyst in hyoid bone: unusual location. J Laryngol Otol 2003; 117(8): 656–657

Definition

▶ **Epidemiology**
No sex predilection • Incidence corresponds to the underlying disease or injury.

▶ **Etiology, pathophysiology, pathogenesis**
Unilateral atrophy of individual muscles or muscle groups due to loss of innervation • *Possible causes:* Trauma, iatrogenic (postoperative or postirradiation), tumor.

– *Mandibular nerve* (cranial nerve V3): Medial and lateral pterygoid muscles, masseter.
– *Mylohyoid nerve* (branch of cranial nerve V3): Mylohyoid muscle, anterior belly of digastric muscle.
– *Facial nerve* (cranial nerve VII): Facial muscles.
– Hypoglossal nerve (cranial nerve XII): Lingual muscles, geniohyoid muscle.

Imaging Signs

▶ **Modality of choice**
MRI, CT.

▶ **CT findings**
Decreased volume of the muscle belly • Possible fat-equivalent attenuation values.

▶ **MRI findings**
Atrophic muscle can be seen on MRI much earlier than CT • Even in the acute or subacute stage (24–48 hours) the affected muscles show an edema-like T2-weighted signal increase with slight swelling • In the chronic stage, the muscles show decreased volume and fatty degeneration (high T1- and T2-weighted signal intensity) • Diagnosis may warrant cranial nerve examination • Comparison of the two sides is helpful.

▶ **Selected normal values**
Transverse diameter of the masseter muscle:
– *In men:* 11–13 mm relaxed, 14–17 mm contracted.
– *In women:* 9–11 mm relaxed, 12–14 mm contracted.

▶ **Pathognomonic findings**
Streaky increase in T1-weighted signal intensity and decreased volume affecting characteristic muscles or muscle groups due to chronic fatty degeneration following denervation.

Clinical Aspects

▶ **Typical presentation**
Symptoms depend on the underlying disease or injury • Rapid fatigue of masticatory muscles • Dysphagia • Facial asymmetry • Deviation of the protruded tongue toward the atrophic side.

Fig. 7.5 Atrophy of the anterior belly of the digastric and mylohyoid muscles on the left side. Plain T1-weighted MR image. The platysma appears as a thin, hypointense line caudal to the fat-replaced muscles. Cause: iatrogenic injury to the mylohyoid nerve, which arises from the mandibular nerve before it enters the mandibular canal.

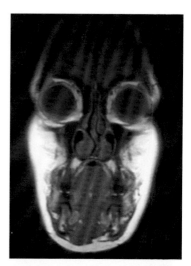

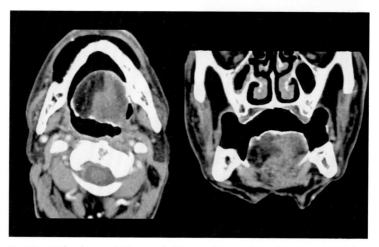

Fig. 7.6 Axial and coronal CT scans of a 71-year-old man who underwent right-sided neck dissection for oropharyngeal carcinoma 10 years earlier. The hypodense fatty area in the right side of the tongue is a result of denervation and irradiation.

▶ **Treatment options**

Treatment of the cause whenever possible: Decompression ● Surgical tumor removal ● Radiotherapy ● Chemotherapy ● Adjunctive measures such as speech therapy, masticatory training, and swallowing exercises.

▶ **Course and prognosis**

Acute muscle changes due to pressure-induced neuropathy are potentially reversible ● Fatty degeneration of muscle is irreversible.

Differential Diagnosis

Neoplasm	– May show similar acute or subacute denervation phase
	– More likely to show diffuse or irregular contrast enhancement
Cellulitis	– Increased extramuscular signal intensity and contrast enhancement
	– "Dirty fat" surrounding the muscle
Fasciitis	– Intense contrast enhancement at the periphery of muscles
Myositis	– Signal characteristics similar to acute or subacute denervation
	– Intense contrast enhancement
	– Stronger perifocal reaction

Tips and Pitfalls

A common error is diagnosing a mass lesion in the healthy, larger muscle.

Selected References

Chang PC, Fischbein NJ, McCalmont TH, Kashani-Sabet M, Zettersten EM, Liu AY, Weissman JL. Perineural spread of malignant melanoma of the head and neck: clinical and imaging features. AJNR Am J Neuroradiol 2004; 25(1): 5–11

King AD, Ahuja A, Leung SF, Chan YL, Lam WW, Metreweli C. MR features of the denervated tongue in radiation induced neuropathy. Br J Radiol 1999; 72(856): 349–353

Russo CP, Smoker WR, Weissman JL. MR appearance of trigeminal and hypoglossal motor denervation. AJNR Am J Neuroradiol 1997; 18(7): 1375–1383

Definition

▶ **Epidemiology**
May occur at any age ● Males predominantly affected ● Often an incidental find-ing ● Maxilla affected more often than the mandible ● Peak incidence at 30–50 years of age.
  – *Follicular cyst:* Seventy-five percent occur in the mandible ● Peak incidence at 30–40 years of age.
  – *Keratocyst:* These form 3–11% of odontogenic cysts ● 66% in the mandible ● Peak incidence at 20–30 years of age.

▶ **Etiology, pathophysiology, pathogenesis**
Uni- or multilocular cystic cavities in the upper or lower jaw ● Derived from den-tal tissues ● Fluid-filled or semisolid ● May have an epithelial lining.
WHO classification:
  – *Type A (inflammatory):* Radicular or residual cyst.
  – *Type B (dysontogenic, odontogenic):* Keratocyst, gingival cyst, follicular cyst.
  – *Types C–E:* classified as nonodontogenic cysts.

Imaging Signs

▶ **Modality of choice**
MRI, CT.

▶ **CT findings**
  – *Radicular cyst:* Apical location ● Rounded oval shape ● Smooth, sclerotic mar-gins.
  – *Follicular cyst:* Develops on the crown of an unerupted tooth ● Unilocular, osteolytic.
  – *Keratocyst:* Located in the mandibular ramus ● May be associated with an unerupted tooth ● Uni- or multilocular ● Sclerotic rim ● Hyperdense.

▶ **MRI findings**
  – *Radicular cyst:* High or low T2-weighted signal intensity ● Enhancing ● May cause root resorption.
  – *Follicular cyst:* High T2-weighted signal intensity ● Rarely causes tooth resorp-tion.
  – *Keratocyst:* Hyperintense to heterogeneous signal intensity on T2-weighted images ● Aggressive ● Does not cause tooth resorption.

▶ **Pathognomonic findings**
None ● Even cysts with a typical appearance require histologic confirmation.

Clinical Aspects

▶ **Typical presentation**
Usually an incidental finding ● Intra- or extraoral swelling ● Inflammation or pain ● Loosening, displacement, or loss of teeth.

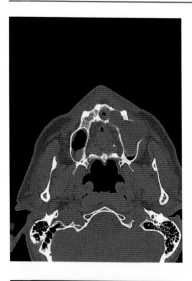

Fig. 7.7 Odontogenic radicular cyst. Plain CT with a bone window shows a thin, smooth, epithelium-lined cyst with marginal sclerosis. Gradual growth has caused the displacement and resorption of adjacent bony structures. The lateral wall of the maxillary sinus appears bowed out due to "inside to outside" growth.

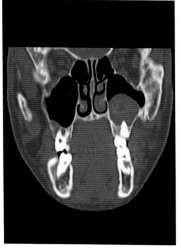

Fig. 7.8 Odontogenic radicular cyst. Plain CT with a bone window. The well-circumscribed cyst has a very thin wall and has expanded within the left maxillary sinus. The cyst contents are isodense to soft tissue. The apex of the root of associated tooth is typically found within the cyst sac.

– *Radicular cyst:* Inflammatory ● Persists or develops after tooth extraction or pulpitis ● Some lesions become symptomatic due to growth or root resorption.
– *Follicular cyst:* Maxillary or mandibular deformity ● Risk of pathologic fracture.
– *Keratocyst:* Maxillary or mandibular deformity ● Aggressive growth with risk of pathologic fracture ● Rarely causes resorption of adjacent teeth.

▶ **Treatment options**
Cystectomy or cystostomy ● Extraction or apical root resection of affected teeth may be required.

▶ **Course and prognosis**
Surgical treatment is curative ● Incidental findings do not require follow-up ● Keratocysts have a 20–60% recurrence rate after surgical removal.

Differential Diagnosis

Neoplasms: ameloblastoma, adenoid carcinoma, mucoepidermoid carcinoma	– Usually associated with extracystic tissue – May also develop in the wall of follicular cysts – Pronounced vestibulolingual extent, resorptive changes
Nonodontogenic cysts, epithelial: nasolabial cyst, incisive canal cyst	– Incisive canal cyst: located between the incisors and nasal floor, smooth margins – Nasolabial cyst: extraosseous, maxillary, close to nasal floor – Postoperative maxillary cyst: history, shows homogeneous resorption
Nonodontogenic cysts, nonepithelial: aneurysmal or simple bone cyst	– Simple or solitary bone cyst: isodense with fluid, smooth walls – Aneurysmal bone cyst: heterogeneous multicystic appearance with fluid–fluid level – Stafne cyst located on lingual side of mandibular angle, thick walls – Rare periapical giant cell tumors

Tips and Pitfalls

Up to 40% of benign tumors are misdiagnosed as simple cysts.

Selected References

Kress G, Gottschalk A, Schmitter M, Sartor K. Benigne Erkrankungen des Unterkiefers im MRT. Fortschr Röntgenstr 2004; 176(4): 491–499
Regezi JA. Odontogenic cysts, odontogenic tumors, fibroosseous, and giant cell lesions of the jaws. Mod Pathol 2002; 15(3): 331–341
Yoshiura K, Weber AL, Runnels S, Scrivani SJ. Cystic lesions of the mandible and maxilla. Neuroimaging Clin N Am 2003; 13(3): 485–494

Definition

▶ **Epidemiology**
Usually of odontogenic or tonsillar origin ● Origin of secondary abscesses can be identified in only 50% of cases.

▶ **Etiology, pathophysiology, pathogenesis**
Circumscribed inflammation of the oral cavity or masticator compartment with liquefaction.
   – *Odontogenic:* Primary extension is usually buccal (to masseter muscle), sublingual, and submandibular ● Extension to palate, oral cavity, or face is less common ● Secondary spread is to para- and retropharyngeal ("danger space") and mediastinal spaces ● Frequently caused by β-hemolytic streptococci.
   – *Tonsillar cause:* Primary extension to the masticator space, medial pterygoid muscle, and soft palate ● Secondary sites same as odontogenic.

Imaging Signs

▶ **Modality of choice**
CT, MRI.

▶ **CT findings**
Asymmetrical soft-tissue mass with ill-defined margins infiltrating adjacent structures ● Frequent uni- or multilocular liquefaction ● Marked enhancement after contrast administration, sometimes with a ring pattern ● Frequently associated cervical lymphadenitis.

▶ **MRI findings**
High T2-weighted signal intensity ● Low T1-weighted signal intensity ● Intense enhancement after gadolinium administration, especially in fat-suppressed sequences ● Rim enhancement with ill-defined margins ● Mandibular osteomyelitis marked by bone-marrow edema and intramedullary enhancement.

▶ **Pathognomonic findings**
Streaky imbibition of the subcutaneous fat ● Liquefaction ● Typical clinical course ● Accompanying apical root abscess, especially in molars ● Mandibular bone destruction due to concomitant osteomyelitis.

Clinical Aspects

▶ **Typical presentation**
Frequent history of dental pain or treatment ● Inflammatory signs (fever, elevated CRP and ESR) ● Most patients have trismus and limited mouth opening ● Facial induration ● Frequent history of ineffectual oral antibiotics.

▶ **Treatment options**
Incision and drainage, needle aspiration ● I.v. antibiotics (e.g., penicillin) indicated for concomitant osteomyelitis.

Fig. 7.9 Contrast-enhanced CT scan of an abscess on the right side of the floor of the mouth, with submandibular extension. The abscess is abutting the right side of the body of the mandible, appearing as a centrally hypodense mass with a ring-enhancing wall. The submandibular gland is displaced posteriorly by the intact wall of the abscess cavity (but is not infiltrated in this case).

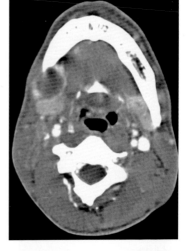

Fig. 7.10 Right paramedian abscess in the floor of the mouth. Postcontrast CT shows the typical centrally hypodense mass with a ring-enhancing wall. A small abscess on the left side is in direct contact with the neurovascular sheath, with associated swelling of the left submandibular soft tissues.

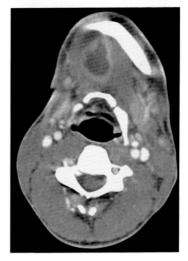

▶ **Course and prognosis**

Good prognosis following incision and drainage and i.v. antibiotics • Rarely, reintervention may be necessary for further drainage • Untreated cases may develop secondary abscess, cellulitis, necrotizing fasciitis or mediastinitis.

Differential Diagnosis

Cellulitis	– Diffuse, enhancing tissue infiltration – No ring-enhancing abscess wall
Tumors (mainly fibrosarcoma and rhabdomyosarcoma)	– Sharper margins with little or no perifocal reaction – Hyperdense, hyperintense, conspicuous mass effect, destructive changes
Unilateral muscular hypertrophy	– Muscle enlargement without typical enhancement after contrast administration

Tips and Pitfalls

An early tumor stage may resemble an abscess on CT and MRI without contrast administration.

Selected References

Bratton TA, Jackson DC, Nkungula-Howlett T, Williams CW, Bennett CR. Management of complex multi-space odontogenic infections. J Tenn Dent Assoc 2002 Fall; 82(3): 39–47

Jones KC, Silver J, Millar WS, Mandel L. Chronic submasseteric abscess: anatomic, radiologic, and pathologic features. AJNR Am J Neuroradiol 2003; 24(6): 1159–1163

Obayashi N, Ariji Y, Goto M, Izumi M, Naitoh M, Kurita K, Shimozato K, Ariji E. Spread of odontogenic infection originating in the maxillary teeth: computerized tomographic assessment. Oral Surg Oral Med Oral Pathol Oral Radiol Endod 2004; 98(2): 223–231

Definition

▶ **Epidemiology**
Children, adolescents, and young adults are predominantly affected • Second peak > 50 years • Acute phase 1–2 weeks, subacute 3–4 weeks • Chronic osteomyelitis is present for at least one month • Chronic cases may be primary, without an acute phase, or may develop secondarily after a maximum of one month • Maxilla is rarely affected (1–6% of cases).

▶ **Etiology, pathophysiology, pathogenesis**
Inflammation of the mandibular bone marrow, sometimes involving the cortex and periosteum • Usually caused by an acute periapical infection or dental pulp infection • Less common causes are mandibular fracture, osteoradionecrosis, and SAPHO syndrome • Immunocompromised patients are predisposed (e.g., HIV infection, steroids, diabetes, tuberculosis, leukemia).

Imaging Signs

▶ **Modality of choice**
MRI, CT.

▶ **CT findings**
Acute phase: Initial signs are demineralization and foci of medullary osteolysis that usually begin distally • Rapid medial progression • Cortical thinning or fistulation • Swelling of surrounding soft tissues common.
Chronic: Subperiosteal spread • Increasing sclerosis and periosteal calcifications (> 80% buccal) • Possible development and demarcation of a sequestrum.

▶ **MRI findings**
  – *Acute phase:* Sensitive detection of bone-marrow edema (high T2-weighted signal intensity, low T1-weighted signal intensity) • Medullary enhancement after gadolinium administration in fat-suppressed T1-weighted sequences • Infiltration of the masseter or medial pterygoid muscle in 30–70% of cases.
  – *Chronic:* Sclerosis may cause decreased signal intensity • Regression of edema and enhancement after contrast administration.

▶ **Pathognomonic findings**
Intraosseous air inclusions • Acute phase: Concomitant apical root abscess • Chronic: Increasing sclerosis of the medullary cavity.

Clinical Aspects

▶ **Typical presentation**
Inflammatory signs (fever, elevated CRP and ESR) • Frequent history of dental pain of treatment (usually acute or chronic secondary) • Trismus usually present • Facial induration • Limited mouth opening • Possible purulent drainage and sinus tract formation.

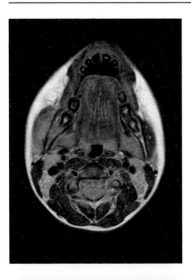

Fig. 7.11 Chronic osteomyelitis of the right hemimandible. Plain axial T2-weighted MR image shows thickening of the body and ramus relative to the opposite side. The bone marrow shows diffuse low signal intensity due to chronic sclerosis and superimposed edema. The right masseter muscle is swollen, and the muscle tissue shows increased signal intensity on the mandibular side.

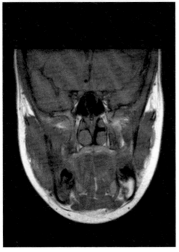

Fig. 7.12 Plain coronal T1-weighted MR image of chronic osteomyelitis of the right hemimandible (same patient as in Fig. 7.**11**). Because of inflammatory edema, the bone marrow in the affected part of body and ramus shows markedly decreased signal intensity compared with the left side. There is associated swelling of the right masseter muscle.

▶ **Treatment options**
  - *Acute phase:* I.v. antibiotics (e.g., penicillin) ● Drainage of abscesses.
  - *Chronic osteomyelitis:* May require surgical debridement of sequestra ● Hyperbaric oxygen therapy may be a helpful adjunct.
▶ **Course and prognosis**
  Good prognosis with specific antibiotic therapy and adequate drainage ● Following surgical debridement, usually bone reconstruction will be needed and facial plastic surgery may be needed ● MRI is recommended for long-term follow-up.

Differential Diagnosis
....

Fibrous dysplasia	– More pronounced expansion, ground-glass opacity (CT)
	– Mixed pattern of nonenhancement and intense enhancement
	– MRI: Patchy T1-weighted signal intensity (hypo- to hyperintense)
Neoplasms (e.g., Ewing sarcoma, osteosarcoma, chondrosarcoma, fibrosarcoma, rhabdomyosarcoma)	– Sharply circumscribed lesion with little or no perifocal reaction
	– Usually causes greater mass effect with a "floating tooth"
	– Periosteal reaction also occurs but is usually spiculated
Metastases	– Typical "moth-eaten" osteolytic pattern
	– Little or no perifocal reaction
Osteoradionecrosis	– Painful bone necrosis, sometimes with sequestration, following radiotherapy

Tips and Pitfalls
....

Histologic confirmation of the diagnosis is advised.

Selected References

Lew DP, Waldvogel FA. Osteomyelitis. Lancet 2004; 364(9431): 369–379
Reinert S, Fürst G, Lenrodt J et al. Die Wertigkeit der Kernspintomographie in der Diagnostik der Unterkiefer-Osteomyelitis. Dtsch Z Mund Kiefer Gesichtschir 1995; 19: 15–18
Schuknecht B, Valvanis A. Osteomyelitis of the mandible. Neuroimag Clin N Am 2003; 13(3): 605–618

Definition

▶ **Epidemiology**
Most common odontogenic tumor (18–35%) ● 81% occur in the mandible, 19% in the maxilla ● Males and females affected equally ● Peak incidence: 30–50 years of age ● 1% of all jaw tumors.

▶ **Etiology, pathophysiology, pathogenesis**
Synonym: Adamantinoma ● Epithelial odontogenic tumor arising from the ameloblasts (innermost layer of the enamel epithelium) ● 1% undergo malignant transformation to ameloblastic carcinoma.

Imaging Signs

▶ **Modality of choice**
CT, MRI.

▶ **CT findings**
Usually multilocular in the mandible, unilocular in the maxilla ● Locally invasive growth ● Small cystic or expansile lesion in the mandibular body and ramus ● Mixed cystic/solid appearance ● Penetrates the cortex ● "Bubblelike" or honeycomb pattern of enhancing intramural papillae ● Periosteal ossification.

▶ **MRI findings**
Well-circumscribed intraosseous mass with intermediate T1-weighted signal intensity ● The high T2-weighted signal intensity of large, expansile ameloblastomas helps in differentiating from malignant tumors ● Desmoplastic type has ill-defined margins.

▶ **Pathognomonic findings**
Even a typical presentation requires histologic confirmation.

Clinical Aspects

▶ **Typical presentation**
Hard, painless tumor mass ● Usually located at the mandibular angle ● Slow growth, often over a period of years ● Frequently associated tooth loss or displacement ● Association with unerupted wisdom teeth.

▶ **Treatment options**
Surgical removal ● Larger lesions should be fully excised by an en-bloc resection ● Curettage, chemotherapy, and radiotherapy are contraindicated.

▶ **Course and prognosis**
Surgical removal is curative ● Unilocular form has a 15% recurrence rate after surgical removal ● Multilocular form (in older patients) has a 33% recurrence rate ● DD: Fibrous union.

Fig. 7.13 Ameloblastoma in the right side of the mandible. Contrast-enhanced CT with a soft-tissue window shows an expansile, bubblelike tumor that has transgressed the midline of the jaw, causing displacement and resorption of the mandibular cortex. The tumor tissue appears isointense to muscle after contrast administration.

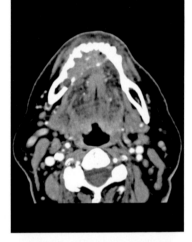

Fig. 7.14 Contrast-enhanced CT with a bone window shows extreme thinning and oral displacement of the cortical bone boundary (same patient as in Fig. 7.**13**). Rarefaction of the cortical bone is also noted in the vestibular area. The tumor tissue contains scattered cortical remnants with osseous density.

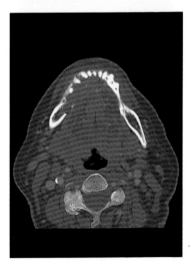

Differential Diagnosis

Radicular cyst	– No enhancing intramural papillae
	– Most are unilocular
	– Widening of the periodontal space
Follicular cyst	– No enhancing intramural papillae
	– Most are unilocular
	– Surrounds the crown of an unerupted tooth
Keratocyst	– No enhancing intramural papillae
	– Most are unilocular or multilocular
	– Often associated with an unerupted tooth
Aneurysmal bone cyst	– Usually large and expansile with heterogeneous, multicystic appearance
	– Multilocular fluid–fluid levels
	– Occurs predominantly in children

Tips and Pitfalls

A small ameloblastoma may be mistaken for a radicular cyst or keratocyst.

Selected References

Manor Y, Mardinger O, Katz J, Taicher S, Hirshberg A. Peripheral odontogenic tumours: differential diagnosis in gingival lesions. Int J Oral Maxillofac Surg 2004; 33(3): 268–273

Minami M, Kaneda T, Yamamoto H et al. Ameloblastoma in the maxillomandibular region: MR imaging. Radiology 1992; 184: 389–393

Wiseman SM, Rigual NR, Alberico RA, Sullivan MA, Loree TR. Ameloblastoma of the mandible. J Am Coll Surg 2003; 196(4): 654

Definition

▶ **Epidemiology**
More common in males (3:1 ratio) ● Peak incidence at 45–60 years of age ● 90% of all oral malignancies are squamous cell carcinomas, 10% are adenocarcinomas ● 90% of lingual carcinomas are located on the border of the tongue, 8% at the base, 2% in the tip ● 20–30% undergo early metastasis to level I and II lymph nodes.

▶ **Etiology, pathophysiology, pathogenesis**
Malignant tumor of the tongue, usually squamous cell carcinoma ● Multifactorial extrinsic (e.g., tobacco, alcohol, viruses) and intrinsic causes (e.g., iron deficiency anemia, age, syphilis, weakened immune status) ● Initial lesion is commonly leukoplakia, followed by dysplasia, carcinoma in situ, and finally invasive carcinoma.

Imaging Signs

▶ **Modality of choice**
MRI, CT.

▶ **CT findings**
Asymmetry of the body of the tongue ● Displacement of the lingual septum ● Loss of normal muscle pennation ● Invasive tumor with necrotic areas, slightly hyperdense to the fatty lingual muscles ● Inhomogeneous enhancement after contrast administration ● Invasion of the mandible and floor of the mouth ● Frequent involvement of ipsilateral cervical lymph nodes ● (Dental) artifacts can be minimized by angulation.

▶ **MRI findings**
Inhomogeneous low T1-weighted signal intensity and high T2-weighted signal intensity in axial, coronal, and sagittal images ● *Artifacts:* See Carcinoma of the Floor of the Mouth ● Enhancement after gadolinium administration.

▶ **Pathognomonic findings**
Invasive mass of the body of the tongue that enhances after contrast administration.

Clinical Aspects

▶ **Typical presentation**
Early stage is usually asymptomatic, appearing as indurated lesion with associated neck pain ● Later stages characterized by tongue fixation due to muscle invasion ● Dysphagia ● Odynophagia and speech impairment ● Oral leukoplakia in approximately a third of cases.

▶ **Treatment options**
Stage T1 or T2: Complete tumor excision with or without mandibular osteotomy ● Glossectomy ● Advanced stages require neck dissection and radiochemotherapy.

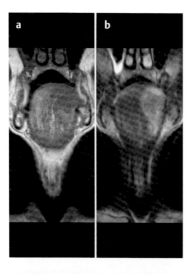

Fig. 7.15 a, b Carcinoma of the tongue. Plain T1-weighted MR image (**a**) and fat-suppressed sequence (**b**) after gadolinium administration. Unenhanced image (**a**) shows squamous cell carcinoma involving the middle to anterior third of the tongue body on the left side. The tumor shows low T1-weighted signal intensity and has not transgressed the midline. The tumor shows intense enhancement after gadolinium administration (**b**). The postcontrast study defines the true extent of the carcinoma, which is extending into the glossoalveolar sulcus.

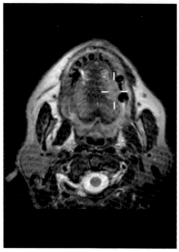

Fig. 7.16 Squamous cell carcinoma of the tongue. Plain T2-weighted MR image. Located in the anterior two-thirds of the left border of the tongue, the tumor (crosshairs) is isointense to muscle on the unenhanced T2-weighted image. The normal pennate pattern of the lingual muscles is absent within the tumor.

► **Course and prognosis**

Five-year survival rate after complete tumor resection is 73–97% ● Larger tumors have a 40% recurrence rate, with up to a 40% incidence of cervical (often bilateral) metastases.

Differential Diagnosis

Tonsillar hyperplasia	– Tonsils usually show symmetrical, homogeneous enlargement – No invasive growth – Enhancing septa
Non-Hodgkin lymphoma	– Unilateral tumor mass with submucous spread – Pronounced, nonnecrotizing lymph node enlargement
Benign salivary gland tumors	– Smooth tumor margins – Sometimes pedunculated – No enhancing septa
Adenoid cystic carcinoma of the minor salivary glands	– Morphologically similar to squamous cell carcinoma – Ill-defined margins – Lymph node metastases are rare
Kaposi sarcoma	– AIDS-associated neoplasia – Mucosal growth similar to squamous cell carcinoma

Tips and Pitfalls

Carcinoma of the body of the tongue may be missed on plain CT scans ● Mass effect or asymmetry may erroneously be attributed to swallowing.

Selected References

Lam P, Au-Yeung KM, Cheng PW, Wei WI, Yuen AP, Trendell-Smith N, Li JH, Li R. Correlating MRI and histologic tumor thickness in the assessment of oral tongue cancer. AJR Am J Roentgenol 2004; 182(3): 803–808

Pimenta Amaral TM, Da Silva Freire AR, Carvalho AL, Pinto CA, Kowalski LP. Predictive factors of occult metastasis and prognosis of clinical stages I and II squamous cell carcinoma of the tongue and floor of the mouth. Oral Oncol 2004; 40(8): 780–786

Weber AL, Romo L, Hashmi S. Malignant tumors of the oral cavity and oropharynx: clinical, pathologic, and radiologic evaluation. Neuroimaging Clin N Am 2003; 13(3): 443–464

Definition

▶ **Epidemiology**
More common in males (3:1 ratio) ● 90% of tumors are squamous cell carcinomas ● Most common tumor of the mandible (by secondary invasion) ● Lymph node metastases in 30–60% of cases.

▶ **Etiology, pathophysiology, pathogenesis**
Malignant tumor of the mucosa of the oral floor ● Multifactorial extrinsic (e.g., 15 times higher incidence with tobacco and alcohol misuse, viral infections) and intrinsic causes (e.g., malnutrition, iron deficiency anemia, age, weakened immune status) ● Begins with dysplasia, progressing to carcinoma in situ and finally invasive cancer.

Imaging Signs

▶ **Modality of choice**
MRI, CT

▶ **CT findings**
Asymmetrical mass in the floor of the mouth ● Isodense or slightly hyperdense to muscle ● Modest enhancement after contrast administration ● Larger tumors may contain necrotic areas and cause bone destruction ● Ipsilateral involvement of submandibular and jugulodigastric lymph nodes ● (Denture) artifacts can be minimized by angulation.

▶ **MRI findings**
Inhomogeneous low T1-weighted signal intensity ● Slightly increased T2-weighted signal intensity ● Soft-tissue and bone-marrow infiltration can be accurately evaluated in axial, coronal, and sagittal images ● Minor denture-related artifacts ● Enhancement after gadolinium administration is clearly appreciated in fat-suppressed sequences.

▶ **Pathognomonic findings**
Sublingual, mucosa-associated tumors that have invaded the oral floor muscles or the mandible are almost always carcinomas.

Clinical Aspects

▶ **Typical presentation**
Leukoplakic lesions in approximately one-third of cases ● 10% of these are carcinoma in situ or invasive squamous cell carcinoma ● Otherwise, initial change consists of slightly raised erythematous area ● Soft, painful tumor is suggestive of perineural spread ● Most tumors are hard and painless, often associated with persistent neck pain, pharyngitis, and otitis media ● Patients are often aware of oral lesion 4–8 months before seeking medical attention.

▶ **Treatment options**
Early stage treatable by complete tumor excision ● Advanced stages require radical tumor excision and neck dissection supplemented by radiochemotherapy.

Fig. 7.17 Oral floor carcinoma next to the left inferior border of the tongue. Contrast-enhanced CT. The obstructed glossoalveolar sulcus is hyperdense relative to the opposite side.

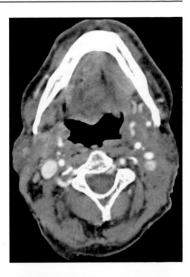

Fig. 7.18 a, b Contrast-enhanced CT. The sublingual squamous cell carcinoma has infiltrated the lingual muscles and shows homogeneous enhancement after contrast administration. Loss of pennation is noted in the genioglossus muscles. The coronal image (**a**) shows the tumor located to the right of the midline above the genioglossi. The sagittal image (**b**) shows the mucosa-associated tumor with invasion of the intrinsic lingual muscles (crosshairs).

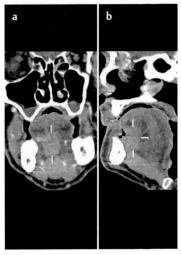

▶ **Course and prognosis**

Prognosis depends on primary tumor size, distant metastases, and particularly on the extent of intra- and extranodal metastases ● T3 and T4 tumors have a three times higher rate of recurrence.

Differential Diagnosis

Benign salivary gland tumors	– Smooth tumor margins – Sometimes pedunculated – No enhancing septa
Malignant tumors of minor salivary glands	– Adenoid cystic carcinoma, morphologically similar to squamous cell – Lymph node metastasis is absent or much less frequent
Kaposi sarcoma	– AIDS-associated neoplasm – Mucosal growth, minimally invasive

Tips and Pitfalls

A common error is to miss a second, latent neoplasm (e.g., bronchial carcinoma). These second tumors are often responsible for existing nodal or distant metastases in patients with a first or early oral squamous cell carcinoma.

Selected References

Weber AL, Bui C, Kaneda T. Malignant tumors of the mandible and maxilla. Neuroimaging Clin N Am 2003; 13(3): 509–524

Weber AL, Romo L, Hashmi S. Malignant tumors of the oral cavity and oropharynx: clinical, pathologic, and radiologic evaluation. Neuroimaging Clin N Am 2003; 13(3): 443–464

Wenzel S, Sagowski C, Kehrl W, Metternich FU. Prognostischer Einfluss der Infiltrationstiefe von Mundhöhlen- und Oropharynxkarzinomen. HNO 2004; 52(7): 604–610

Anatomy

▶ **Parotid gland.**
The parotid gland is located on the masseter muscle anteroinferior to the external auditory canal in the retromandibular fossa. It is bounded superiorly by the zygomatic arch and medially by the pterygoid muscles, styloid process, internal and external carotid arteries, and internal jugular vein. It is bounded posteriorly by the sternocleidomastoid muscle and the posterior belly of the digastric. The parotid duct (Stensen duct) pierces the masseter muscle and opens in the buccal mucosa opposite the second upper molar. The facial nerve enters the parotid gland lateral to the posterior part of the digastric and divides into its main branches within the gland.

▶ **Submandibular gland.**
The submandibular gland is located in the submandibular fossa medial to the mandible, lateral to the digastric, and below the mylohyoid, which separates the submandibular space from the sublingual space above it. Its excretory duct (submandibular duct, Wharton duct) opens in the sublingual caruncle, often accompanied by the small ducts of the sublingual gland.

▶ **Sublingual gland.**
The sublingual gland is located in the floor of the mouth below the sublingual fold.

▶ **Minor salivary glands.**
Besides the three paired major salivary glands, there are several hundred minor salivary glands distributed in the mucosa of the palate, pharynx, cheek, and lips.

Definition

▶ **Epidemiology**
  – *Aplasia of the salivary glands or duct system:* Rare • Combined with aplasia of the lacrimal glands and ducts in 38% of cases.
  – *Accessory elements of the parotid gland:* Normal variant in 20% of cases.
  – *Muscular anomalies in the parotid region:* Inferior auricular muscle, occipito-parotid muscle (extremely rare).

▶ **Etiology, pathophysiology, pathogenesis**
  – *Accessory salivary gland tissue:* Results from inclusions in lymph nodes or the abnormal descending migration of salivary gland tissue.
  – *Muscular anomalies:* Fan-shaped expansion of muscle fibers blending with the parotid fascia.
  – *Hypoplasia and aplasia of major salivary glands:* Result from abnormal development of the ectoderm of the first and second branchial arches (ectodermal dysplasia) • Often combined with other symptom complexes: Levy–Hollister syndrome, EEC (ectrodactyly-ectodermal dysplasia-clefting) syndrome, Treacher Collins syndrome (mandibulofacial dysostosis) • Some cases have an autosomal dominant inheritance.

Imaging Signs

▶ **Modality of choice**
  MRI.

▶ **CT findings**
  Absent glandular tissue replaced by hypodense fat in the gland bed • Ectopic glandular tissue appears as a lobulated, uniformly hyperdense, well-circumscribed mass that enhances after contrast administration.

▶ **MRI findings**
  Absence of glandular tissue with T1- and T2-weighted hyperintense fat in the gland bed • Accessory glandular tissue appears on T1-weighted images as a sharply circumscribed, lobulated mass hyperintense to muscle • MRI is superior to CT for demonstrating the glandular tissue.

▶ **Pathognomonic findings**
  – *Accessory salivary glands:* Usually distributed along the Stensen duct in the upper and lower nuchal region, especially about the sternocleidomastoid and masseter muscles • Rare: Pituitary, middle ear, external auditory canal, mandible, thyroid capsule, lymph nodes • Diameter 3 cm or less • Drainage from the main gland into the Stensen duct.
  – *Choristoma:* Ectopic salivary gland tissue in the gingiva or middle ear.
  – *Salivary gland aplasia:* Absence of one or more salivary glands • Gland bed usually occupied by fatty tissue with hypertrophy of other salivary glands.

Fig. 8.1   Accessory submental salivary gland. Incidental CT finding in a woman with a cystic mass in the right side of the neck.

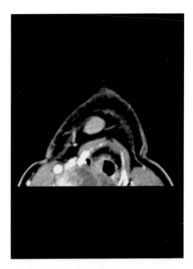

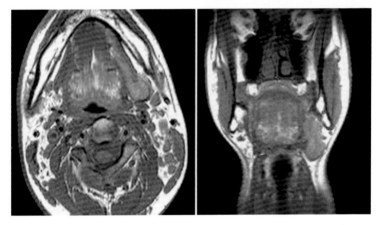

Fig. 8.2   Aplasia of the right submandibular gland with fat in the gland bed (axial and coronal T1-weighted MR image).

Clinical Aspects

▶ **Typical presentation**
- *Aplasia:* Unilateral aplasia of the major salivary glands is usually asymptomatic (incidental finding, palpable asymmetry) • Bilateral aplasia of the parotid gland may lead to hyposalivation • Absence of all four major salivary glands causes xerostomia with eating and swallowing difficulties • Premature caries.
- *Levy–Hollister syndrome:* Xerostomia • Sensorineural hearing loss • Auricular dysmorphia • Keratoconjunctivitis (aplasia of lacrimal ducts).
- *Accessory salivary gland tissue:* Often an incidental finding • Symptoms usually result from inflammatory or neoplastic complications.

▶ **Treatment options**
Surgical resection of ectopic salivary gland tissue when complications arise (mucocele, fistulation, tumor, abscess) • Xerostomia treatable with artificial saliva, copious oral fluids, and improved dental hygiene.

▶ **Course and prognosis**
Of all parotid gland tumors, 1–7% develop from accessory glandular tissue, especially pleomorphic adenoma and mucoepidermoid carcinoma.

▶ **What does the clinician want to know?**
Diagnosis • With ectopic tissue: Location, signs of benignancy or malignancy, possibility of diagnostic needle biopsy.

Differential Diagnosis

Salivary gland tumors	– Suspicion raised by palpable asymmetry and hyperplasia of the unaffected gland
	– Easily differentiated by MRI and CT, which show fat replacement of glandular tissue in aplasia and ectopic glandular tissue with an accessory gland

Tips and Pitfalls

Ectopic tissue may raise false suspicion of a tumor or metastasis • Tissue sampling is important in confirming the diagnosis.

Selected References

Chilla R, Steding G. Über Muskelanomalien in der Regio parotidea – ein Beitrag zur Parotischirurgie. Laryngo-Rhino-Otol 2001; 80: 748–749

Fierek O et al. Das Levy-Hollister-Syndrom: Ein Dysplasiesyndrom mit HNO-Manifestationen. HNO 2003; 51: 654–657

Goldenberg D et al. Misplaced parotid glands: Bilateral agenesis of parotid glands associated with bilateral accessory parotid tissue. J Laryngol Otol 2000; 11: 883–887

Definition

▶ **Epidemiology**
Second most common tumor of the parotid gland (12%) • Accounts for 5% of all salivary gland tumors • More common in males (3:1) • Average age of occurrence is 60 years • Bilateral in 10–15% of cases • 20% multicentric • Greatly increased risk in smokers.

▶ **Etiology, pathophysiology, pathogenesis**
Cystadenolymphoma • Tumor develops from lymphatic tissue that is deposited in the parotid gland during embryonic development.

Imaging Signs

▶ **Modality of choice**
MRI.

▶ **CT findings**
Complex internal structure with hypodense, cystic, multilocular components • Faint to intense enhancement after contrast administration.

▶ **MRI findings**
Usually iso- to hypointense on T1-weighted images • Areas of high T1-weighted signal intensity represent protein-rich or hemorrhagic cysts • Intermediate to high T2-weighted signal intensity • Moderate enhancement after gadolinium administration.

▶ **Pathognomonic findings**
Usually located in the posterior superficial part of the parotid gland • Sharply circumscribed inhomogeneous mass • 30% have a cystic appearance • Papillary nodular thickening in the cyst wall • No calcifications.

Clinical Aspects

▶ **Typical presentation**
Well-circumscribed mass below the earlobe • May have fluid consistency • Painless.

▶ **Treatment options**
Tumor resection with healthy margins, preserving the facial nerve.

▶ **Course and prognosis**
Recurrence rate is uncertain due to multicentricity and frequent presence of other small nodular lesions in the gland.

▶ **What does the clinician want to know?**
Diagnosis • Tumor extent • Signs of malignancy in equivocal cases.

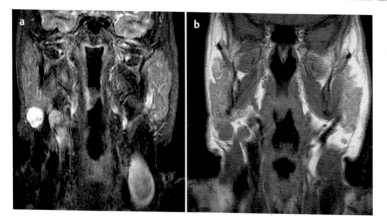

Fig. 8.3 a, b Warthin tumor. Coronal STIR sequence (**a**) shows a hyperintense mass at the inferior pole of the right parotid gland. In the T1-weighted image (**b**), the mass is hypointense to glandular tissue.

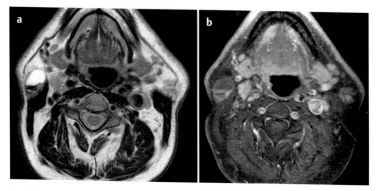

Fig. 8.4 a, b In axial sequences the anterior cystic component of the mass shows high T2-weighted signal intensity (**a**) and low T1-weighted signal intensity after gadolinium administration (**b**). The solid posterior component enhances in the T1-weighted image (**b**).

Differential Diagnosis

Pleomorphic adenoma	– Sharply circumscribed tumor with intense but inhomogeneous enhancement after contrast administration – May contain calcifications – Large tumors are often lobulated with a pear-shaped configuration and extension into deep part of gland
Mucoepidermoid carcinoma	– Firm, painful mass – Frequent facial nerve paralysis – Poorly delineated from surroundings – Early lymph node metastases – Some tumors are cystic with necrotic and hemorrhagic foci
Lymphoma	– Rare – Circumscribed enhancement with intraparotid nodular lymph node involvement – Diffuse enhancement with parenchymal involvement
Lymphoepithelial cysts	– Usually present in HIV – Sharply circumscribed, homogeneous, cystic mass with a thin wall – Frequently bilateral

Tips and Pitfalls

Small lesions are difficult to distinguish from mucoepidermoid carcinoma • Small multicentric or contralateral lesions may be missed.

Selected References

Harnsberger HR. Handbook of Head and neck imaging. St Louis: Mosby; 1995

Minami M et al. Warthin tumor of the parotid gland: MR-pathologic correlation. AJNR 1993; 14: 209–214

Shugar JM, Som PM, Biller HF. Warthin's tumor, a multifocal disease. Ann Otol Rhinol Laryngol 1982; 91: 246–249

Definition

▶ **Epidemiology**
Highest incidence at approximately 30 years of age ● 50% of patients give a history of trauma to the mandible or nuchal region.

▶ **Etiology, pathophysiology, pathogenesis**
Retention cyst of the sublingual gland or minor salivary glands ● Usually acquired (postinflammatory, posttraumatic), rarely congenital.
  – *Simple ranula:* Retention cyst lined by sublingual space epithelium due to duct obstruction ● Respects fascial boundaries of the submandibular space.
  – *Diving (complicated) ranula:* Results from rupture of the capsule with extension into the submandibular space ● Pseudocyst without an epithelialized wall ● May extend into the prestyloid parapharyngeal space.

Imaging Signs

▶ **Modality of choice**
MRI.

▶ **MRI findings**
Sharply circumscribed homogeneous mass ● Low T1-weighted signal intensity with wall enhancement after gadolinium administration ● High T2-weighted signal intensity ● Diving ranula appears on T2-weighted images as a hyperintense fluid rim around the posterior border of the mylohyoid muscle ● Inflammation leads to wall thickening.

▶ **CT findings**
Hypodense sublingual mass with an enhancing wall.

▶ **Pathognomonic findings**
  – *Simple ranula:* Unilocular oval mass in the sublingual space.
  – *Diving ranula:* Comet-tail-shaped mass with the "tail" in the collapsed sublingual space and "head" in the posterior submandibular space ● Thin fluid rim between the mylohyoid muscle and the hyoglossus or geniohyoid.

Clinical Aspects

▶ **Typical presentation**
Tense, painless swelling of the sublingual gland (elevation of the tongue tip) ● Bluish discoloration.

▶ **Treatment options**
Extirpation of the sublingual gland.

▶ **Course and prognosis**
Gradual enlargement of the untreated simple ranula with eventual rupture and progression to a diving ranula ● Resection is curative.

▶ **What does the clinician want to know?**
Usually a clinical diagnosis ● Extension into the submandibular space?

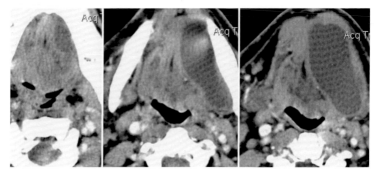

Fig. 8.5 Ranula. Axial CT scans show a sharply marginated, hypodense mass in the left sublingual and submandibular area with expansion of the sublingual gland.

Differential Diagnosis

Epidermoid cyst	– Indistinguishable from a simple ranula
	– Unlike a diving ranula, has no perimylohyoid fluid rim
Dermoid	– Mass of variable density and signal intensity due to varying tissue components
Cystic hygroma	– Has same MRI signal characteristics but usually shows multilocular spread
	– No fluid rim in the submandibular space
Retention cyst of submandibular gland	– Cyst in the submandibular space, no cyst in the sublingual space

Tips and Pitfalls

Some ranulas are difficult to visualize due to artifacts from teeth or dental fillings •
A complicated ranula with a collapsed "tail" may be mistaken for a retention cyst of the submandibular gland.

Selected References

Coit WE et al. Ranulas and their mimics: CT evaluation. Radiology 1987; 163: 211–216
Kurabayashi T et al. MRI of ranulas. Neuroradiology 2000; 42: 917–922
Macdonald AJ et al. Giant ranula of the neck: differentation from cystic hygroma. Am J Neuroradiol 2003; 24(4): 757–761

Definition

▶ **Epidemiology**
Sialolithiasis: 30–60/1 million • 2200–5000 new cases per year.

▶ **Etiology, pathophysiology, pathogenesis**
Sialadenitis: Inflammation of a major salivary gland • Sialolithiasis: Stone in a salivary gland or its excretory duct.
Acute sialadenitis: Usually an ascending infection (streptococci, staphylococci) • Causes: Decreased salivation (dehydration, decreased food intake), weakened immune status, salivary stones • Rare: Hematogenous spread, drug-induced.
Epidemic parotitis (mumps): Viral cause • 85% in children • Bilateral involvement in 75% of cases.
Chronic recurrent parotitis: Often related to an immunologic disorder • Genetic predisposition • Malformation of the parotid gland • Impaired production of secretions leading to duct obstruction.
Radiation sialadenitis: Radiation doses ≥6 Gy induce gland swelling • Doses ≥15 Gy damage the gland parenchyma • Doses ≥40 Gy cause parenchymal atrophy.
Sialolithiasis: Most common in the fifth to eighth decades • 80% in the submandibular gland • 15% in the parotid gland • Multiple stones in 7–13% • Combination of calcium phosphate compounds and phospholipids or proteolipids • Microliths generated by autophagocytosis of calcium-rich cellular organelles with stenosis and ductectasia • Associated with sialadenitis in 50% of cases • 10–20% of stones are nonradiopaque.

Imaging Signs

▶ **Modality of choice**
  – *Acute sialadenitis:* Sonography • Sialography is contraindicated (may exacerbate the inflammation).
  – *Chronic sialadenitis:* (MR) sialography.
▶ **Sonographic findings**
  – *Acute sialadenitis:* Hypoechoic gland • Color duplex sonography shows hyperemia • Possible air inclusions.
  – *Chronic sialadenitis:* Inhomogeneous echo pattern • Hypoechoic cystlike areas represent foci of ductectasia.
  – *Sialolithiasis:* Hyperechoic complex with a posterior acoustic shadow • Stones <2 mm may be nonshadowing.
▶ **Sialographic findings**
  – *Chronic sialadenitis:* Irregular ductectasia or alternating duct expansion and stenosis.
  – *Sialolithiasis:* Concave filling defect caused by the stone • Possible prestenotic ductectasia • Contrast medium must be free of air bubbles (to avoid spurious findings).

Fig. 8.6 Sialolithiasis. Axial CT scan demonstrates a small, sharply circumscribed, hyperdense nodule in the left parotid gland.

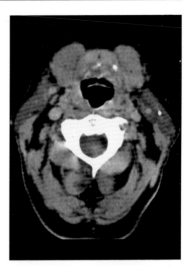

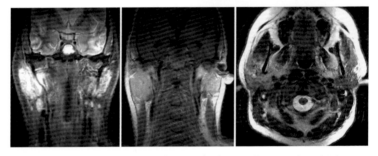

Fig. 8.7 Coronal STIR image and axial T2-weighted image show an enlarged right parotid gland with inhomogeneous low signal intensity. Coronal T1-weighted image shows only moderate enhancement of the gland after gadolinium administration consistent with chronic sialadenitis (left: coronal STIR image; center: postcontrast coronal T1-weighted image; right: axial T2-weighted image).

▶ **CT findings**
- *Sialadenitis:* Enlarged gland • Indistinct margins • Gland is hypodense on plain scans and shows greater enhancement after contrast administration than the healthy opposite gland • Abscesses are hypodense and sometimes loculated.
- *Sialolithiasis:* Plain thin-slice CT is most sensitive for stone detection • Hyperdense, sharply circumscribed nodule.

▶ **MRI findings**
- *Acute sialadenitis:* Indistinct margins • High T2-weighted signal intensity • Low T1-weighted signal intensity • Marked enhancement after gadolinium administration • Unsharpness and expansion of the surrounding fat and masseter muscle with increased T2-weighted signal intensity.
- *Chronic sialadenitis:* Inhomogeneous signal with low T1-weighted signal intensity and high to intermediate T2-weighted signal intensity • Long-standing cases often show glandular atrophy with decreased signal intensity.
- *Radiation sialadenitis:* Atrophy • Inhomogeneous signal • MR sialography shows foci of ductectasia and abrupt caliber changes in larger ducts.
- *Sialolithiasis:* Sharply circumscribed discontinuity in the duct (with low T2-weighted signal intensity).

▶ **Pathognomonic findings**
- *Acute sialolithiasis:* Swollen gland with convex lateral surface.
- *Chronic sialadenitis:* Frequent atrophy, but gland size is variable.
- *Sialolithiasis:* Most stones are 6–8 mm in diameter, with a maximum size of 50 mm • CT shows a hyperdense nodule in the gland or duct.

Clinical Aspects

▶ **Typical presentation**
Acute sialadenitis: Pain and swelling • Fever • Papillary redness • Swelling of the excretory duct • Purulent saliva reflects bacterial etiology • Most common in elderly and immunocompromised patients.
Chronic recurrent parotitis: Ten times more prevalent in adults • Women are predominantly affected (but most affected children are males) • Recurrent episodes of moderately painful parotid swelling of several days' duration • Flocculent, salty saliva.
Radiation sialadenitis: Decreased salivation (hypoptyalism).
Sialolithiasis: Postprandial swelling of the gland with tension pain • Eventual permanent enlargement due to secondary inflammation.

▶ **Treatment options**
Acute sialadenitis: Antibiotics (cephalosporins) • Anti-inflammatory agents • Antipyretics • Stimulation of salivation (chewing gum, citrus drops, lemons, ascorbic acid lozenges) • Abscesses treated by incision and drainage.
Chronic recurrent parotitis: Antibiotics in the acute phase • Anti-inflammatory agent • (Sub)total parotidectomy with ligation of the excretory duct close to the papilla.

Radiation sialadenitis: Stimulation of salivation ● Anti-inflammatory agents ● Artificial saliva.

Sialolithiasis: Balloon catheter insertion to dilate the duct ● Intraoral surgery with incision of the anterior part of the excretory duct ● Deep-sited stones can be removed by external surgery ● Ultrasound lithotripsy.

▶ **Course and prognosis**
  – *Acute sialadenitis:* Rare cases develop necrotizing fasciitis or necrotizing otitis externa.
  – *Viral sialadenitis (mumps):* Risk of meningitis, pancreatitis, and orchitis.
  – *Radiation sialadenitis:* Possible xerostomia ● Prophylactic administration of cytoprotective agents (Amifostine).
  – *Chronic recurrent parotitis:* Parotidectomy permanently relieves complaints in 80–100% of cases ● Risk of facial nerve injury at operation.
  – *Sialolithiasis:* 50–100% success rate, depending on cause and therapeutic approach.

▶ **What does the clinician want to know?**
Diagnosis ● Stone detection and localization in patients with sialolithiasis.

Differential Diagnosis

Sjögren syndrome	– Bilateral, inhomogeneous weblike pattern – Small- to medium-sized nodularity of the parenchyma – Decreased echogenicity
Sialadenosis	– Swelling of parotid gland – Rarefied, narrowed duct system with homogeneous parenchyma – "Leafless tree" pattern
Sarcoidosis	– Cervical and mediastinal lymph node involvement – Parotid swelling with cystic/solid changes – Enhancement of granulomas after contrast administration

Tips and Pitfalls

Air bubbles inadvertently injected during sialography may be misinterpreted as sialolithiasis.

Selected References

Gritzmann N et al. Sonography of the salivary glands. Eur Radiol 2003; 13 (5): 964–975

Maier H. Therapie nichttumoröser Speicheldrüsenerkrankungen und postoperativer Komplikationen. Laryngo-Rhino-Otol 2001; 80 (1): 89–114

Yousem DM et al. Major salivary gland imaging. Radiology 2000; 216: 19–29

Zenk Z, Iro H. Die Sialolithiasis und deren Behandlung. Laryngo-Rhino-Otol 2001; 80 (1): 115–136

Definition

▶ **Epidemiology**
Incidence of 5/1000 per year ● Second most common rheumatic disease (after rheumatoid arthritis) ● More common in females (9:1) ● Association with HLA DR2 and DR3.

▶ **Etiology, pathophysiology, pathogenesis**
Synonym: Myoepithelial sialadenitis ● Autoimmune dysfunction leads to destruction of acinar cells and ductal epithelial cells of the salivary and lacrimal glands by infiltrating activated lymphocytes.
  – *Type I:* Primary form ● Unknown etiology.
  – *Type II:* Secondary form ● "Sicca syndrome" in rheumatoid arthritis, collagen diseases, hepatitis C, primary biliary cirrhosis.

Imaging Signs

▶ **Modality of choice**
MRI, MR sialography.

▶ **MRI findings**
Diffuse (honeycomb), bilateral low T1-weighted signal intensity ● With severe fibrosis there is less enhancement after gadolinium administration ● Strong enhancement after gadolinium administration reflects high clinical activity ● High T2-weighted signal intensity ● Classification:
  – Stage I: Enhancement after gadolinium administration, high T2-weighted signal intensity ≤ 1 mm.
  – Stage II: Enhancement after gadolinium administration, high T2-weighted signal intensity 1–2 mm.
  – Stage III: Enhancement after gadolinium administration, high T2-weighted signal intensity > 2 mm.
  – Stage IV: Destruction of glandular parenchyma.

▶ **CT findings**
Hypodense (fluid-isodense) diffuse lesions with variable-size cysts and honeycombing, depending on the stage ● Clear delineation of calcium-dense stones.

▶ **Sialographic and MR sialographic findings**
Multiple punctate foci of enhancement after gadolinium/contrast administration ● Mixed pattern of lobular, cavitary, and destructive involvement ● Enlarged parotid gland with honeycomb pattern ● Ectasia and stenosis of excretory ducts.

▶ **Sonography**
Fibrotic parenchymal changes ● Decreased echogenicity.

▶ **Pathognomonic findings**
Swollen parotid gland with small- to medium-sized nodularity and honeycombing of the parenchyma ● Increasing fibrosis over time ● Tendency for stone formation.

Fig. 8.8 Sjögren syndrome. Contrast-enhanced CT shows bilateral inhomogeneous parenchymal density in both glands and decreased gland size as a result of fibrosis.

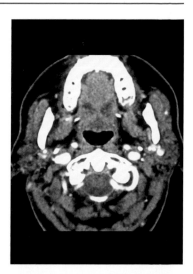

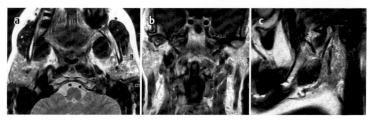

Fig. 8.9 a–c Same patient as Fig 8.8. MR images in all three planes show inhomogeneous glandular tissue, especially in the left parotid gland, with small cystic areas of high T2-weighted signal intensity (**a**).

Clinical Aspects

▶ **Typical presentation**

Predominantly affects middle-aged and older women ● Painless swelling of the salivary glands ● "Sicca syndrome": Keratoconjunctivitis sicca with dry eyes (xerophthalmia) and dry mouth (xerostomia).

  – Laboratory tests: SS-B antibodies, SS-A antibodies (70%) ● Rheumatoid factors (50%) ● Positive Schirmer test ● Biopsy of inner lip ● Secondary forms associated with symptoms of underlying disease (e.g., arthritis, scleroderma).

▶ **Treatment options**

Treatment of underlying disease in secondary cases ● Chewing gum to promote salivary gland activity ● Artificial saliva ● Eyedrops ● Increased fluid intake ● bromhexine (promotes secretion) ● Surgical treatment for abscess formation.

▶ **Course and prognosis**

Primary type is most common and takes a benign course ● Malignant lymphoma (NHL) develops in 4–8% of cases (p. 196) ● Prognosis of secondary type depends on underlying disease ● *Complications:* corneal ulceration; rare cases develop vasculitis and renal or pulmonary involvement.

▶ **What does the clinician want to know?**

Diagnosis ● Remaining "viable" glandular tissue ● Foci of duct stenosis.

Differential Diagnosis

Sarcoidosis	– Cervical and mediastinal lymph nodes
	– Parotid swelling with cystic/solid changes
	– Enhancement of granulomas after contrast administration
Benign lymphoepithelial cysts in HIV	– Parotid swelling
	– Multiple cystic lesions with a thin wall
	– Possible cervical lymphadenopathy
Warthin tumor	– May be bilateral
	– Well-delineated cystic/solid mass with nodular thickening of the cyst wall
	– Usually located in posteroinferior part of gland
Sialadenosis	– Parotid swelling
	– Rarefied, narrowed duct system with homogeneous parenchyma

Tips and Pitfalls

May be confused with sialadenosis ● Air bubbles inadvertently injected during sialography can mimic stenotic lesions of the parotid duct.

Selected References

Izumi M et al. MR imaging of the parotid gland in Sjogren's syndrome: a proposal for new diagnostic criteria. AJR 1996; 166: 1483–1487

Ohbayashi N et al. Sjogren syndrome: comparison of assessments with MR sialography and conventional sialography. Radiology 1998; 209: 683–688

Tonami H et al. MR sialography in patients with Sjogren syndrome. AJNR Am J Neuroradiol 1998; 19: 1199–1203

Definition

▶ **Epidemiology**

Occurs predominantly in the parotid gland, occasionally in the submandibular gland • Males and females affected equally • No peak age incidence, but slightly more common after 40 years of age • *Predisposing factors:* Weakened host defenses, dehydration, addiction (e.g., alcohol, heroin, barbiturates), ductectasia, duct obstruction.

▶ **Etiology, pathophysiology, pathogenesis**

Develops in a setting of sialadenitis (usually an ascending inflammation) • Main causative organisms: *Staphylococcus aureus*, streptococci, peptostreptococci, mycobacteria • Submandibular and sublingual gland abscesses may be secondary to dental or alveolar crest infections (e.g., after tooth extraction).

Imaging Signs

▶ **Modality of choice**

Sonography, CT, MRI to investigate equivocal findings or complications.

▶ **Sonographic findings**

Enlarged gland with a hypoechoic structure • Mass with well-defined or ill-defined margins • Echo-free center, often with posterior acoustic enhancement • Fresh abscess may contain internal echoes • Thin abscess membranes often cannot be visualized with ultrasound.

▶ **CT findings**

Enlarged, hypodense gland with increased enhancement after contrast administration • Hypodense mass with an enhancing membrane • May contain air inclusions • Possible duct stones.

▶ **MRI findings**

Enlarged gland • Poorly demarcated mass with increased T2-weighted signal intensity and marked enhancement after gadolinium administration • High T2-weighted signal intensity, low T1-weighted signal intensity, rim-enhancing membrane after gadolinium administration • Susceptibility artifacts may result from gas inclusions.

▶ **Pathognomonic findings**

Expansion of the salivary gland • Liquid mass, usually elliptical, with well- or ill-defined margins and an enhancing membrane • May contain air inclusions • Usually associated with edematous expansion of the buccal fat pad, subcutaneous fat, and masseter muscle.

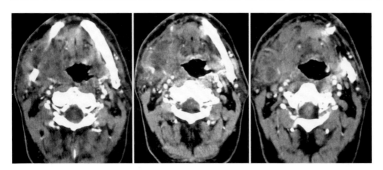

Fig. 8.10 Salivary gland abscess. CT demonstrates a large mass with indistinct margins, a hypodense center, and an enhancing membrane in the right submandibular area. Increased density of the adjacent fat signifies an inflammatory perifocal reaction.

Clinical Aspects

▶ **Typical presentation**
Very painful swelling and redness of the salivary gland with a feeling of tension ● Definite fluctuation typical of an abscess is seen in only 30% of cases ● Leukocytosis ● Fever.

▶ **Treatment options**
Peri- and postoperative i.v. antibiotics (first and second generation cephalosporins) ● Anti-inflammatory agents ● Analgesics ● Abscess drainage with facial nerve monitoring and wound irrigation (hydrogen peroxide) ● Excisional biopsy and smear should be obtained for confirmation ● Multiple abscesses may necessitate parotidectomy.

▶ **Course and prognosis**
Postoperative course is usually good ● In chronic recurrent parotitis abscesses may recur after treatment.

▶ **What does the clinician want to know?**
Diagnosis ● Extent of the abscess ● Duct stones.

Differential Diagnosis

Warthin tumor	– 30% have a cystic appearance with papillary-nodular thickening of the cyst wall – Inhomogeneous internal structure – Faint to marked enhancement after contrast administration
Mucoepidermoid carcinoma	– Firm painful mass, often with associated facial paralysis – Poorly demarcated from surroundings – Early lymph node metastases – Mixed cystic, necrotic, and hemorrhagic pattern
Lymphoepithelial cysts	– Most common in HIV patients – Sharply circumscribed, homogeneous, cystic mass with a thin wall – Frequently bilateral
Metastases	– Peri- or intraparotid lymph node metastases arising from ENT malignancy or malignant melanoma – Frequently multiple, often have a necrotic center – Painless

Tips and Pitfalls

Some abscesses are difficult to distinguish from mucoepidermoid carcinoma ● Reactive lymph node enlargement may be misinterpreted as metastases.

Selected References

Gritzmann N et al. Sonography of the salivary glands. Eur Radiol 2003; 13: 964–975
Thiede O et al. Klinische Aspekte der abszedierenden Parotitis. HNO 2002; 50: 332–338
Yousem DM et al. Major Salivary Gland Imaging. Radiology 2000; 216: 19–29

Definition

▶ **Epidemiology**
80% of all parotid tumors ● Other salivary glands are involved in 20–30% of cases (6.5% submandibular gland, 6.5% minor salivary glands) ● Most common in middle age (30–60 years) ● 2:1 female preponderance ● 5% rate of malignant transformation.

▶ **Etiology, pathophysiology, pathogenesis**
Benign tumor of myoepithelial origin ● Arises from distal part of parotid duct system including intervening ducts and acini ● Slow-growing parotid tumor with variegated epithelial histology.

Imaging Signs

▶ **Modality of choice**
MRI.

▶ **CT findings**
Hyperdense to surrounding salivary gland tissue on plain scans ● Postcontrast CT shows intense, often inhomogeneous tumor enhancement with hypodense areas (necrosis or retained mucus) ● Occasional calcifications.

▶ **MRI findings**
Hyperintense mass on T2-weighted images ● Low to intermediate signal intensity on T1-weighted and PD-weighted images ● Areas with high T1-weighted signal intensity are due to hemorrhage ● Homogeneous to inhomogeneous enhancement (necrosis) after gadolinium administration, depending on lesion size.

▶ **Pathognomonic findings**
Sharply circumscribed elliptical mass, usually located in the posteroinferior part of the parotid gland ● Small adenomas usually have homogeneous parenchyma surrounded by parotid tissue ● Large adenomas are often lobulated with a pear-shaped configuration and indent the parapharyngeal space ● Larger tumors have a more complex parenchymal structure with necrotic, hemorrhagic, or calcified areas.
Special form: Iceberg tumor (synonym: dumbbell tumor) ● Dumbbell-shaped extension through the parapharyngeal space into the tonsillar fossa.

Clinical Aspects

▶ **Typical presentation**
Buccal (preauricular) mass, usually painless ● Smooth, solid, well demarcated and clearly palpable ● Pressure from constant growth causes atrophy of the surrounding tissue ● Salivation is usually not impaired ● Pressure-induced facial nerve paralysis is rare.

▶ **Treatment options**
Surgical removal of the entire tumor, preferably with a margin of glandular tissue to prevent recurrence ● Radiotherapy is recommended for elderly patients with tumor encasing the facial nerve.

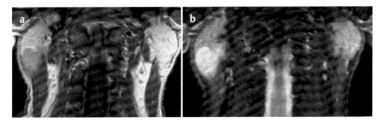

Fig. 8.11 a, b Pleomorphic adenoma. T1-weighted image (**a**) shows a sharply circumscribed, hypointense mass at the inferior pole of the right parotid gland. The tumor shows high signal intensity in the STIR sequence (**b**).

Fig. 8.12 In a T1-weighted image with fat suppression, the posteriorly situated mass shows marked, somewhat inhomogeneous enhancement after gadolinium administration.

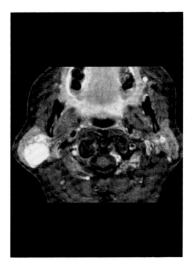

► **Course and prognosis**
Tumors recur in 5% of cases ● 5% undergo malignant transformation (most common with frequently recurring tumors).

► **What does the clinician want to know?**
Diagnosis ● Tumor extent ● Facial nerve changes.

Differential Diagnosis

Warthin tumor	– Bilateral in some cases – Well-delineated cystic/solid mass with nodular thickening of the cyst wall – Usually located in the posteroinferior part of the gland
Adenoid cystic carcinoma	– Diffuse, infiltrative pattern of spread – Early facial paralysis – Frequent erosion of the retromandibular vein
Mucoepidermoid carcinoma	– Firm, painful mass – Frequent facial paralysis – Poorly demarcated from surroundings – Early lymph node metastasis – Mixed cystic, necrotic, and hemorrhagic pattern

Tips and Pitfalls

Because of their inhomogeneous structure, large adenomas are difficult to distinguish from malignant tumors. Closely scrutinize the deep portion of the parotid gland!

Selected References

Ikeda et al. The usefulness of MR in establishing the diagnosis of parotid pleomorphic adenoma. AJNR 1996; 17: 555–559

Phillips PP et al. Recurrent pleomorphic adenoma of the parotid gland: report of 125 cases and a review of the literature. Ann Otol Rhinol Laryngol 1995; 104: 100–141

Som PM et al. Benign and malignant parotid pleomorphic adenomas: CT and MR studies. J Comput Assist Tomogr 1988; 12: 65–69

Definition

▶ **Epidemiology**
4–5% of all extranodal lymphomas occur in the salivary glands • Account for 3.7% of all parotid gland tumors • 70% in the parotid gland • 40% of NHL cases in children show parotid gland involvement • 4–8% of patients with Sjögren syndrome (p. 187) develop a lymphoma.

▶ **Etiology, pathophysiology, pathogenesis**
Most salivary gland lymphomas are of the non-Hodgkin type • Most occur in a setting of HIV infection, systemic dissemination, or chronic myoepithelial parotitis (Sjögren syndrome) • Most lesions (50%) are MALT lymphomas • Usually arise from intraglandular lymph nodes • Extranodal involvement in 40% of cases.

Imaging Signs

▶ **Modality of choice**
MRI.

▶ **MRI findings**
Salivary gland mass with a nodular or diffuse configuration • Iso- to hypointense on T1-weighted images • Iso- to hyperintense on T2-weighted images • Moderate enhancement after gadolinium administration.

▶ **CT findings**
Nodular mass, usually with cervical lymphadenopathy and moderate enhancement after contrast administration • Parenchymal involvement shows diffuse enhancement after contrast administration.

▶ **Sonographic findings**
Mass hypoechoic to normal glandular tissue • Homogeneous echo pattern in cases with nodal involvement and primary involvement of the parotid gland • Inhomogeneous pattern with secondary involvement.

▶ **Pathognomonic findings**
Nodal involvement: Conglomerate nodal masses displacing the glandular parenchyma and showing small parapharyngeal extensions • *Extranodal involvement:* Diffuse, inhomogeneous glandular swelling, sometimes with interspersed microcystic areas.

Clinical Aspects

▶ **Typical presentation**
Females affected more than males • Peak incidence in the fifth to sixth decade • With nodal involvement, continuous swelling of the gland • With extranodal involvement, recurrent swelling of the gland • Systemic manifestations (fever, night sweats, weight loss) • Rare instances of facial palsy.

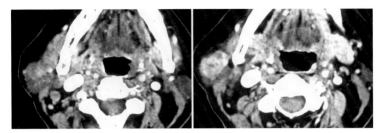

Fig. 8.13 Lymphoma. CT demonstrates enhancing nodular masses in the right parotid gland. The largest lymphomatous focus displays central necrosis.

▶ **Treatment options**
- Extranodal salivary gland involvement: Complete tumor resection followed by radiotherapy.
- Nodal involvement: No benefit from invasive surgery.
- MALT lymphoma: Combination of chemotherapy and radiation.

▶ **Course and prognosis**
Better prognosis with extranodal involvement, with a lower recurrence rate and less frequent disseminated disease ● Nodal involvement has 50% mortality despite treatment ● Five times higher recurrence rate with nodal involvement ● MALT lymphomas have a better prognosis.

▶ **What does the clinician want to know?**
Diagnosis ● Extent of disease ● Signs of nodal or extranodal involvement ● Cervical lymphadenopathy.

Differential Diagnosis

Metastases	– Common with malignant melanoma and squamous cell carcinoma of the skin
	– Possible multifocal occurrence
	– 4.3% of solid parotid tumors
Adenoid cystic carcinoma	– Diffuse, infiltrating pattern of spread
	– Early facial palsy
	– Frequent erosion of retromandibular vein
Carcinoma	– High-grade carcinomas show invasive growth with indistinct margins and inhomogeneous enhancement after contrast administration

Tips and Pitfalls

Nodular involvement is difficult to distinguish from metastasis.

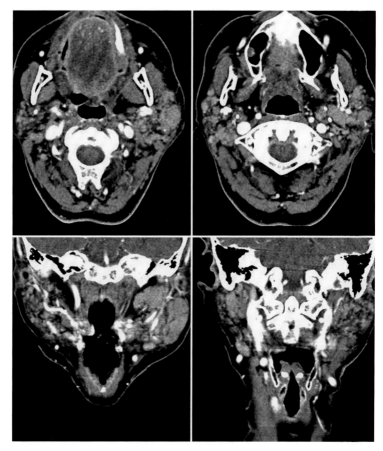

Fig. 8.14   NHL in a 30-year-old man. CT reveals micronodular lymphomatous involvement of the right parotid gland and large nodular foci in the left parotid gland. The scans also show adjacent retromandibular and cervical lymphadenopathy.

Selected References

Jaehne M et al. The clinical presentation of non-Hodgkin lymphomas of the major salivary glands. Acta Orolaryngol 2001; 121: 647–651

Rodriguez M. Computed tomography, magnetic resonance imaging and positron emission tomography in non-Hodgkin's lymphoma. Acta Radiol 1998; 39: 1–36

Tonami H et al. Clinical and imaging findings of lymphoma in patients with Sjögren syndrome. J Comput Assist Tomogr 2003; 27 (4): 517–524

Tonami H et al. Mucosa-associated lymphoid tissue lymphoma in Sjögren's syndrome: Initial and follow-up imaging features. AJR 2002; 179: 485–489

Definition

▶ **Epidemiology**
The smaller the gland, the greater the likelihood that a tumor is malignant:
  – 50–80% occur in the sublingual gland and minor salivary glands (40% muco-epidermoid carcinoma, 40% adenoid cystic carcinoma, 5% acinar cell carcinoma).
  – 40–50% occur in the submandibular gland (mostly adenoid cystic carcinoma).
  – 20–25% occur in the parotid gland (60% mucoepidermoid carcinoma, 15% acinar cell carcinoma, 5% adenoid cystic carcinoma).

▶ **Etiology, pathophysiology, pathogenesis**
Mucoepidermoid carcinoma: Arises from ductal epithelium ● Majority are low-grade, slow-growing malignancies ● Small percentage are high-grade malignancies with rapid growth and early lymphogenous metastasis.
Adenocarcinoma: Slow-growing tumor.
Adenoid cystic carcinoma: Slow-growing tumor, often with perineural spread.
Acinar cell carcinoma: Originates from ductal cells ● Peak incidence in the fourth to fifth decades ● 2:1 female preponderance ● Slow growing ● Bilateral in 3% of cases.
Squamous cell carcinoma: Rare ● Usually develops in a setting of chronic sialadenitis ● Fast growing ● 2:1 female preponderance ● Peak incidence after 60 years of age.
Classification:
  – Stage T1: 2 cm or smaller, no extraparenchymal spread.
  – Stage T2: 2–4 cm, no extraparenchymal spread.
  – Stage T3: > 4 cm and/or extraparenchymal spread.
  – Stage T4a: Invasion of the skin, mandible, external auditory canal, and facial nerve.
  – Stage T4b: Invasion of the skull base, pterygoid process, and internal carotid artery.

Imaging Signs

▶ **Modality of choice**
MRI, CT.
▶ **CT findings**
  – Low-grade carcinoma: Well delineated ● Usually homogeneous tumor showing moderate enhancement after contrast administration.
  – High-grade carcinoma: Invasive growth ● Ill-defined margins ● Inhomogeneous enhancement after contrast administration.
▶ **MRI findings**
High-grade carcinomas show inhomogeneous T2-weighted and T1-weighted signal intensity with inhomogeneous enhancement after gadolinium administration ● High T2-weighted signal intensity comes from cystic and necrotic areas (especially in mucoepidermoid and squamous cell carcinomas) ● Tumor extent is best appreciated on unenhanced T1-weighted images.

Fig. 8.15 • Parotid carcinoma. Axial CT demonstrates a large, solid, strongly enhancing mass in the left parotid gland.

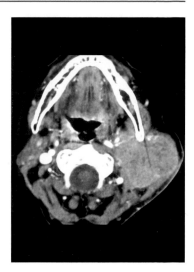

► **Pathognomonic findings**

Most important criterion is invasive growth • Inhomogeneous contrast enhancement • Low-grade malignancies are usually well demarcated from surrounding glandular tissue • Acinar cell carcinoma is usually surrounded by a capsule • Mucoepidermoid carcinoma may contain calcifications and cystic areas • Definitive diagnosis relies on histology.

Clinical Aspects

► **Typical presentation**

Firm swelling of the salivary gland with a variable growth rate • Usually painful (most acinar cell carcinomas are painless) • Frequent facial paralysis (mucoepidermoid carcinoma, adenocarcinoma, squamous cell carcinoma) • Possible associated cranial nerve deficits (third division of trigeminal nerve, especially with adenoid cystic carcinoma).

► **Treatment options**

Tumor resection with clear margins • Acinar cell carcinoma and undifferentiated carcinoma often require total parotidectomy with sacrifice of facial nerve branches or the entire nerve, followed by radiotherapy • Neck dissection for metastases • Primary radiotherapy for inoperable disease.

► **Course and prognosis**

Survival rate depends on tumor grade:
– *Mucoepidermoid carcinoma:* 5-year survival rate is 90% with low-grade carcinoma, 40% with high-grade carcinoma • Recurrence rate is 15%.

- *Adenocarcinoma:* Early facial palsy ● Often infiltrates the retromandibular vein, later invading the pterygoid muscles and internal carotid artery.
- *Adenoid cystic carcinoma:* 10-year survival rate is approximately 65% ● Early facial palsy ● Regional lymph node metastases are rare ● Hematogenous metastasis to lung and bone.
- *Squamous cell carcinoma:* Extensive regional lymph node involvement and distant metastases are usually present at time of diagnosis.
- *Acinar cell carcinoma:* Hematogenous metastasis to lung and bone plus regional lymph node metastases.

▶ **What does the clinician want to know?**
Intra- or extraparenchymal growth ● Lymph node metastases ● Distant metastases ● Perineural growth pattern (trace the facial nerve from the stylomastoid foramen).

Differential Diagnosis

Pleomorphic adenoma	– Sharply circumscribed tumor, usually oval, may include necrotic and calcified areas
	– Caution: 5% rate of malignant transformation with rapid tumor growth
Warthin tumor	– Sometimes bilateral
	– Well-delineated cystic/solid mass with nodular thickening of the cyst wall
	– Usually located in the posteroinferior part of the gland
Lymphoma	– Rare
	– Circumscribed enhancement with intraparotid lymph node involvement
	– Diffuse enhancement with parenchymal involvement
Metastases	– Peri- or intraparotid lymph node metastases originating from ENT malignancies or malignant melanoma
	– Often multiple, often with central necrosis

Tips and Pitfalls

A diagnosis of malignancy usually requires histologic confirmation.

Selected References

Casselmann JW, Mancuso AA. Major salivary gland masses: comparison of MR imaging and CT. Radiology 1987; 165: 183–189

Freling NJ et al. Malignant parotid tumors: clinical use of MR imaging and histologic correlation. Radiology 1992; 185: 691–696

Yousem DM et al. Major salivary gland imaging. Radiology 2000; 216: 19–29

Definition

▶ **Epidemiology**
Most common (90–95%) of all branchiogenic malformations (cysts, fistulas) ● Usually clinically silent in newborns ● Often first recognized in adolescents and adults ● Initial diagnosis usually made at 20–40 years of age.

▶ **Etiology, pathophysiology, pathogenesis**
Cyst in the lateral cervical triangle ● Arises from the second (or occasionally the third) branchial arch ● In the sixth week of embryonic development, the second branchial arch overgrows the third and fourth arches and the second through fourth branchial clefts ● Persistent communication results in cysts and fistulas.

Imaging Signs

▶ **Modality of choice**
MRI, CT.

▶ **CT findings**
Cystic mass (10–25 HU) lateral to the neurovascular sheath (up to 10 cm in diameter) ● Displaces the submandibular gland anteromedially, displaces the sternocleidomastoid muscle posterolaterally ● Often located near the mandibular angle; occasionally parapharyngeal or anterior to neurovascular sheath ● Septation and intracystic hemorrhage (density) are rare ● Only infected cysts show enhancement of the thickened wall after contrast administration.

▶ **MRI findings**
T1-weighted signal intensity depends on protein and blood content (low = hypointense, high = hyperintense) ● High T2-weighted signal intensity ● Well-circumscribed, noninfiltrating mass ● Intense enhancement of the wall after gadolinium enhancement is seen only in infected cysts.

▶ **Pathognomonic findings**
Nonenhancing smooth-bordered cyst located medial to the neurovascular sheath, anterior to the sternocleidomastoid muscle, and posterior to the submandibular gland.

Clinical Aspects

▶ **Typical presentation**
Soft, usually asymptomatic mass in the region of the mandibular angle or lateral neck ● May become infected ● Infection characterized by pain and lymph node swelling ● Openings of sinus tracts on the skin surface are visible at birth ● These may drain mucus.

▶ **Treatment options**
Complete cystectomy with adequate margins to remove any sinus tracts.

▶ **Course and prognosis**
Excellent prognosis after complete resection ● Infection hampers surgical removal.

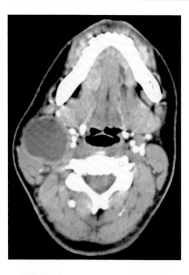

Fig. 9.1 Infected branchial cleft cyst. Postcontrast CT. A cyst at the level of the right mandibular angle shows central low density with a thickened, enhancing wall. The sternocleidomastoid muscle has been displaced posterolaterally and the neurovascular sheath medially.

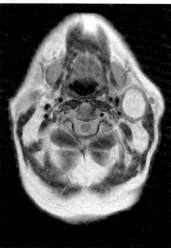

Fig. 9.2 Unenhanced T2-weighted MR image of a branchial cleft cyst in the left submandibular region. The center of the cyst is markedly hyperintense, and the cyst wall shows intermediate signal intensity. The sternocleidomastoid muscle has been displaced posterolaterally, the neurovascular sheath medially.

Differential Diagnosis

Inflammatory or malignant lymph node enlargement	– Central enhancement after contrast administration (in the absence of central necrosis) – Usually multiple, distributed along vessels
Cystic hygroma	– Usually multilocular – Often larger and septated – Most common in children younger than 2 years of age
Abscess	– Usually incites inflammatory reaction in surrounding tissue
Hematoma	– No enhancing wall – Signal changes
Thymic cyst	– Located at a more caudal level and within the neurovascular sheath – Cystic mass, sometimes with a spongelike appearance
Cystic neurinoma	– Lateral to the neurovascular sheath

Tips and Pitfalls

May be confused with abscess or hematoma • Differentiating feature: Relationship to neurovascular sheath.

Selected References

Dernis HP, Bozec H, Halimi P, Vilde F, Bonfils P. Cyst of the parapharyngeal space arising from the branchial arches. Ann Otolaryngol Chir Cervicofac 2004; 121(3): 175–178

Girvigian MR, Rechdouni AK, Zeger GD, Segall H, Rice DH, Petrovich Z. Squamous cell carcinoma arising in a second branchial cleft cyst. Am J Clin Oncol 2004; 27(1): 96–100

Lev S, Lev MH. Imaging of cystic lesions. Radiol Clin North Am 2000; 38(5): 1013–1027

Definition

▶ **Epidemiology**
No sex predilection • Common in the fifth decade • 2–4% due to spontaneous bleeding in response to anticoagulant treatment • Up to 1% of cases result from carotid injury, which is associated with 20–40% mortality.

▶ **Etiology, pathophysiology, pathogenesis**
Bleeding into cervical organ parenchyma, fascial compartments, or soft tissues • More than 40% of cases are iatrogenic (injury, anticoagulation) • 25% are post-traumatic (rupture, fracture) • 5% are inflammatory (erosion) • A few cases are tumor-related (thyroid or parathyroid adenoma) or spontaneous (13% hemorrhagic diathesis and hemophilia; 15% copious vomiting, vigorous coughing or sneezing).

Imaging Signs

▶ **Modality of choice**
CT, MRI.

▶ **CT findings**
Hyperacute to subacute collections appear as a hyperdense mass (40–80 HU) • May be unrelated to organs or other structures • No enhancement after contrast administration except in cases with active bleeding and contrast extravasation.

▶ **MRI findings**
Differentiation of blood breakdown products by stages:
  – Hyperacute and subacute: Increased T2-weighted signal intensity.
  – Acute and chronic: Decreased T2-weighted signal intensity.
  – Hyperacute and acute: Intermediate T1-weighted signal intensity.
  – Subacute: Increased T1-weighted signal intensity.
  – Chronic: Decreased T1-weighted signal intensity.
  – Susceptibility artifacts (blood breakdown products) appear in GE sequences.

▶ **Selected normal values**
Conventional radiographs (sagittal diameter): Prevertebral space 1–7 mm (C2 level), retrotracheal space 9–21 mm (C6 level), laryngeal inlet 15–23 mm, glottic inlet 17–25 mm, trachea 14–20 mm. Widening or displacement is suspicious for hematoma.

▶ **Pathognomonic findings**
Hyperdense cervical mass unrelated to organs • High unenhanced T1-weighted and T2-weighted signal intensity with susceptibility artifacts (blood products) in GE sequences.

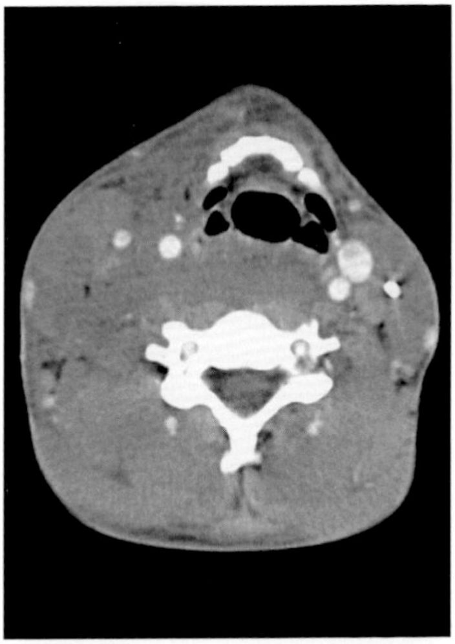

Fig. 9.3 Cervical hematoma. Postcontrast CT shows swelling of the right sternocleidomastoid muscle and displacement of the surrounding fat spaces with no enhancement after contrast administration. The hematoma is isodense to surrounding muscle. There is complete compression of the right internal jugular vein.

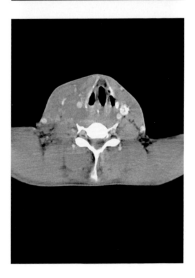

Fig. 9.4 Postcontrast CT (same patient as in Fig. 9.**3**) shows generalized swelling of the cervical soft tissues on the right side with compression of the surrounding structures and asymmetrical displacement of the thyroid cartilage toward the left side.

Clinical Aspects

▶ **Typical presentation**

Symptoms of underlying disease or injury ● Three main symptoms: Airway narrowing (80%), swelling (usually anterior tracheal displacement), visible subcutaneous hematoma in the neck and upper chest ● Hemopneumothorax present in approximately 25% of posttraumatic cases.

▶ **Treatment options**

Intubation or tracheotomy for respiratory distress ● Conservative treatment ● Hemostasis by vascular compression or ligation ● Hematoma evacuation ● Aspiration.

▶ **Course and prognosis**

Prognosis ranges from very good (57%) to grave (22%), depending on the timing of treatment ● Risk of infection after hematoma evacuation.

Differential Diagnosis

Abscess	– Typical intense ring enhancement
Neoplasms	– Enhances after contrast administration, may show central necrosis
	– Usually does not spread along fascial planes
Inflammatory or malignant lymph node swelling	– Usually multiple or conglomerated
	– Enhances after contrast administration
	– Typically rounded shape
	– Does not spread along fascial planes

Tips and Pitfalls

Cervical hematomas are easily missed on posttraumatic CT scans of the cervical spine when attention is focused on the spine itself (using a bone window only).

Selected References

Delank KW. Blutungen im HNO-Bereich: Fachspezifische und interdisziplinare Aspekte. HNO 2005; 53(2): 187–197

Paleri V, Maroju RS, Ali MS, Ruckley RW. Spontaneous retro- and parapharyngeal haematoma caused by intrathyroid bleed. J Laryngol Otol 2002; 116(10): 854–858

White P, Seymour R, Powell N. MRI assessment of the pre-vertebral soft tissues in acute cervical spine trauma. Br J Radiol 1999; 72(860): 818–823

Definition

▶ **Epidemiology**
Virtually all age groups affected ● No sex predilection ● 5% of all thromboses ● Usually iatrogenic (e.g., caused by a catheter, cardiac pacemaker, or irradiation) ● Inflammatory etiology has become rare.

▶ **Etiology, pathophysiology, pathogenesis**
Acute, subacute, or chronic occlusion of the internal jugular vein by thrombosis ● Three causes (Virchow triad):
  – Endothelial defect (e.g., from an indwelling catheter or i.v. drug misuse).
  – Slowing or stasis of blood flow (e.g., due to tumor compression or invasion).
  – Coagulation disorder (e.g., tumor related).

Imaging Signs

▶ **Modality of choice**
CT, MRI.

▶ **CT findings**
Acute and subacute cases usually show an increase in the caliber of the jugular vein with decreased central density (intraluminal thrombus) ● After i.v. contrast administration, opacified blood forms a rim around the thrombus ● Chronic progressive vascular obliteration leads to complete occlusion or collateralization ● Thrombophlebitis is marked by enhancement of the vein wall ● Possible abscess formation.

▶ **MRI findings**
  – *Acute, subacute:* Mass with characteristic blood-thrombus signal characteristics ● Surrounding increase in T2-weighted signal intensity.
  – *Chronic:* Increased T1-weighted signal intensity in the vein ● Decreased T1-weighted signal intensity (blood breakdown).
  – *MRA:* Absent flow signal or intraluminal filling defect.

▶ **Selected normal values**
Normal diameter of internal jugular vein shows high inter- and intraindividual variability ● Right side: 12 mm (range 6–23 mm) ● Left side: 10.5 mm (range 5–19 mm).

▶ **Pathognomonic findings**
(Partially occlusive) thrombus in the lumen of the internal jugular vein.

Clinical Aspects

▶ **Typical presentation**
  – *Incidental finding:* Swelling in the neck ● Lateral, infrahyoid, or supraclavicular.
  – Paraneoplastic (Trousseau syndrome).
  – Tumor-related compression or infiltration.
  – *Acute thrombophlebitis:* Fever ● Soft, painful swelling (DD: abscess) ● Postural guarding ● Rare fulminating sepsis.

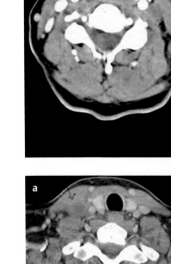

Fig. 9.5 Jugular vein thrombosis. Post-contrast CT. The left internal jugular vein is completely occluded by an older thrombus. The vein diameter is unchanged relative to the opposite side. The lumen is not perfused by the contrast medium and is slightly hypodense to surrounding muscle. Note the increased luminal size of the ipsilateral external jugular vein, which is functioning as a collateral vessel.

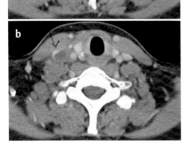

Fig. 9.6 a, b Postcontrast axial CT of a fresh thrombus in the right internal jugular vein (**a**). The vein diameter is increased relative to the opposite side, and the thrombus is markedly hypodense to surrounding muscle tissue. Scan taken at a slightly higher level (**b**) shows a thin, crescent-shaped rim of contrast medium around the thrombus.

Soft Tissues of the Neck

– *Chronic jugular vein thrombosis:* Hard, sometimes painless swelling (DD: neoplasm).

▸ **Treatment options**

Antibiotics (aerobic and anaerobic) for treatment and prevention of infection • Anticoagulants may be given (heparin 30 000 IU/day for 10 days) • Resection or ligation of the vein is rarely indicated, as very few pulmonary emboli are seeded from the upper circulation • Most cases resolve by spontaneous recanalization or collateralization.

▸ **Course and prognosis**

Thrombophlebitis is usually present for up to 2 weeks before thrombosis occurs • Underlying disease is often a limiting factor.

Differential Diagnosis

Abscess	– Rarely tubular – Stronger enhancement after contrast administration – May abut the vein or occur elsewhere
Neoplasm (necrotic)	– Almost never tubular – Usually shows lower T1-weighted signal intensity than thrombosis – May abut the vein or occur elsewhere
Inflammatory or malignant lymph node swelling	– Usually multiple or form a conglomerate mass – Enhancement after contrast administration – Distributed along the vein, which often is normally delineated

Tips and Pitfalls

Acute thrombophlebitis with an enhancing wall may be mistaken for an abscess.

Selected References

Boedeker CC, Ridder GJ, Weerda N, Maier W, Klenzner T, Schipper J. Ätiologie und Management von Thrombosen der Vena jugularis interna. Laryngorhinootologie 2004; 83(11): 743–749

Mamede RC, de Oliveira Resende E Almeida K, de Mello-Filho FV. Neck mass due to thrombosis of the jugular vein in patients with cancer. Otolaryngol Head Neck Surg 2004; 131(6): 968–972

Tajima H, Murata S, Kumazaki T, Ichikawa K, Tajiri T, Yamamoto Y. Successful interventional treatment of acute internal jugular vein thrombosis. AJR Am J Roentgenol 2004; 182(2): 467–469

Definition

▶ **Epidemiology**
Prevalence of 1–5% ● Present in 10–20% of young stroke patients ● Women predominantly affected.

▶ **Etiology, pathophysiology, pathogenesis**
Abnormal expansion or delamination of the ICA wall. Three types of dissection are distinguished: Stenotic, occlusive, and aneurysmal (50%) ● Pseudoaneurysm develops in 25–33% of cases ● Most ICA aneurysms and dissections are extracranial.
– *Aneurysm:* Usually atherosclerotic ● Occasionally traumatic or inflammatory ● Rarely mycotic.
– *Dissection:* Often spontaneous or posttraumatic ● Iatrogenic ● Intrinsic (α-1 antitrypsin deficiency, Marfan and Ehlers Danlos syndromes).

Imaging Signs

▶ **Modality of choice**
MRI/MRA, CT/CTA.

▶ **CT findings**
Aneurysm: Located between the carotid bifurcation and cavernous sinus ● Usually atherosclerosis: Ringlike calcification ● Expansion of the ICA ● Possible atherosclerotic wall changes.
Dissection: Gold standard is intraarterial angiography ● False lumen is hypodense ● Ring pattern of enhancement (vasa vasorum).

▶ **MRI findings**
Aneurysm: Mass with ICA-associated signal loss on T1- and T2-weighted images ● Partial thrombosis with a partial increase in T1-weighted signal intensity ● Fusiform luminal narrowing.
Dissection: Key sequence is T1-weighted with fat suppression ● Eccentric ring with high T1- and T2-weighted signal intensity (intramural hematoma) ● Possible occlusion and central flow void.

▶ **Selected normal values**
Normal diameter of internal carotid artery = 4.6 ± 0.7 mm.

▶ **Pathognomonic findings**
Aneurysm: Flow void within the mass, communicating with the ICA.
Dissection: Intimal septation within the ICA lumen.

Clinical Aspects

▶ **Typical presentation**
Headache ● Tinnitus ● Migraine symptoms and diplopia ● *Aneurysm:* Pulsating parapharyngeal mass ● *Dissection:* TIA, PRIND and stroke symptoms ● Focal neurologic deficit with cranial nerve involvement in 12%, usually affecting CN V and/or combinations, e.g., III, IV and VI (ocular) or IX, X, XI, and XII (lower cranial nerves).

Fig. 9.7 Dissection of the left internal carotid artery just below the skull base. Plain T2-weighted image shows a typical, hyperintense crescent-shaped intramural hematoma involving almost the entire vascular circumference. Residual intraluminal flow appears as a flow void. Fluid retention in the left mastoid (high signal intensity) is noted as an incidental finding.

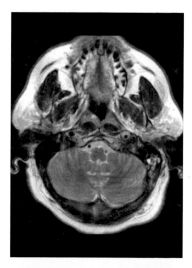

Fig. 9.8 Fat-suppressed T1-weighted image without contrast medium (same patient as in Fig. 9.**7**). The fresh mural hematoma described above is defined even more clearly as an eccentric ring of high signal intensity.

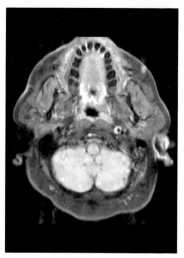

► **Treatment options**

Aneurysm: Operative, angiographic or conservative, depending on location ● Stent insertion may improve the prognosis ● Anticoagulation improves the prognosis.

Dissection: Immediate anticoagulation ● Operative treatment or stent insertion is rarely necessary.

► **Course and prognosis**

Aneurysm: Good prognosis with anticoagulation ● Ruptures are rare.

Dissection: 50% spontaneous resolution rate with anticoagulation ● Recurrence is rare.

Differential Diagnosis

Paraganglioma	– High T2-weighted signal intensity; T1-weighted signal is iso- or hyperintense to muscle – Linear signal voids (as in hemangioma)
Pleomorphic adenoma	– Inhomogeneous – Less distinct margins – Matrix calcifications
Neurinoma, meningioma	– Slower onset of enhancement after contrast administration – Matrix calcifications
Vascular pseudotumors (ectasia, tortuosity, duplication)	– Difficult to delineate, as they are also ICA-associated – Morphology (angiography may advance the DD)

Tips and Pitfalls

An ICA aneurysm that is not definitely excluded by imaging may lead to fatal complications during surgery in the parapharyngeal space.

Selected References

Bakhos D, Lescanne E, Cottier JP, Beutter P, Moriniere S. Extracranial internal carotid artery aneurysm. Ann Otolaryngol Chir Cervicofac 2004; 121(4): 245–248

Jewells V, Castillo M. MR angiography of the extracranial circulation. Magn Reson Imaging Clin N Am 2003; 11(4): 585–597

Pelkonen O, Tikkakoski T, Pyhtinen J, Sotaniemi K. Cerebral CT and MRI findings in cervicocephalic artery dissection. Acta Radiol 2004; 45(3): 259–265

Definition

▶ **Epidemiology**
All age groups are affected ● Often retropharyngeal in children (skull base to T4 vertebra) ● Primary focus cannot be identified in 50% of cases ● β-hemolytic streptococci are often the causative organisms.

▶ **Etiology, pathophysiology, pathogenesis**
Encapsulated (abscess) or nonencapsulated (cellulitis) spread of inflammation ● Contiguous spread of inflammation from the upper respiratory tract (e.g., tonsillitis, pharyngitis, sialadenitis, glossitis) or teeth ● Sometimes there is extracapsular spread of cervical lymphadenitis along the neurovascular sheath or posterior cervical triangle ● Less frequent cause is transjugular i. v. drug abuse.

Imaging Signs

▶ **Modality of choice**
CT, MRI.

▶ **CT findings**
Ill-defined, diffuse obliteration of fat planes (cellulitis) or uni-/multilocular fluid and gas collections with surrounding edema and wall enhancement (abscess) ● May contain serous exudation or pus (density > 30 HU).

▶ **MRI findings**
Fatty tissue infiltration with low T1-weighted and high T2-weighted signal intensity ● Indistinct anatomical boundaries ● Spread along fascial planes, usually down into the mediastinum (cellulitis) ● Abscesses show peripheral rim enhancement and do not respect anatomical boundaries.

▶ **Pathognomonic findings**
Abscess: Mass with enhancing inflammatory rim, may contain small gas–fluid levels.
Cellulitis: Diffuse area of increased density and enhancement distributed along fascial planes.

Clinical Aspects

▶ **Typical presentation**
Over 50% of patients have already received antibiotic therapy at diagnosis for inflammations of the oral cavity (teeth), oropharynx (tonsils), or neck ● Severe neck pain ● Nuchal pain and stiffness ● Fever.

▶ **Treatment options**
Incision and drainage ● High-dose i. v. antibiotics.

▶ **Course and prognosis**
Abscess: Good prognosis after drainage (aspiration) and antibiotics.
Cellulitis: Less favorable prognosis ● Risk of descending necrotizing mediastinitis and fasciitis.

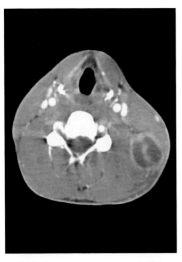

Fig. 9.9 Septic granulomatosis in a 27-year-old man. Postcontrast CT shows a large, rounded abscess with an intensely enhancing rim located posterior to the left sternocleidomastoid muscle. The abscess cavity is hypodense and septated.

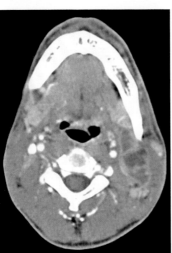

Fig. 9.10 Postcontrast CT scan of a left retromandibular abscess with multiple internal septa at the level of the mandibular angle. The abscess displays a typical pattern of central hypodense (liquid) areas bounded by enhancing walls. The soft tissues surrounding the abscess are swollen.

Soft Tissues of the Neck

Differential Diagnosis

Parapharyngeal inflammation	– Inhomogeneous enhancing fatty tissue ("dirty fat") – No ring-enhancing abscess wall
Primary cysts (branchiogenic, dermoid, epidermoid)	– Often have homogeneous, fluid-equivalent internal structure – Wall enhances only when the cyst is infected
Benign tumor (e.g., adenoma with cystic regressive changes)	– Inhomogeneous internal structure, diffuse contrast enhancement – Smooth outer margins – Low T2-weighted signal intensity, high T2-weighted signal intensity
Carcinomas (mucoepidermoid, adenoid cystic, acinar cell)	– Inhomogeneous internal structure showing diffuse contrast enhancement – Ill-defined margins that do not respect fascial boundaries
Cavitating lymph nodes	– Multiple lymph nodes – Normal fatty tissue

Tips and Pitfalls

The possibility of mediastinal and retropharyngeal spread should always be considered, especially in children.

Selected References

Ashar A. Odontogenic cervical necrotizing fasciitis. J Coll Physicians Surg Pak 2004; 14(2): 119–121

Mihos P, Potaris K, Gakidis I, Papadakis D, Rallis G. Management of descending necrotizing mediastinitis. J Oral Maxillofac Surg 2004; 62(8): 966–972

Zwaan M, Ahrens KH, Blume B. Computerized tomography findings in neck abscess. Laryngorhinootologie 1990; 69(9): 483–485

Definition

▶ **Epidemiology**
Most common form of lymphangioma ● 5% of all benign tumors in newborns and children ● 90% are diagnosed by age 2 years ● Rare in adults ● 68% of affected children have an abnormal karyotype (Turner syndrome, trisomy 21, trisomy 18, trisomy 13).

▶ **Etiology, pathophysiology, pathogenesis**
Cervical lymphangioma with fibrocystic structure ● Develops from primitive lymph sacs of the internal jugular vein ● 80% of hygromas arise from the posterior cervical triangle or lower half of the face, 20% from the axilla, 5% from the mediastinum ● Secondary mediastinal infiltration occurs in 3% ● Most cystic hygromas in adults are in the submandibular, sublingual, or parotid region ● *Structure:* Cysts often contain fibrous septa and serous, protein-rich fluid (lymph) ● Often coexist with other subtypes of lymphangioma (cavernous, capillary) or mixed tumors with hemangiomatous elements.

Imaging Signs

▶ **Modality of choice**
Sonography (especially intrauterine) ● MRI for evaluating soft-tissue infiltration.

▶ **Sonographic findings**
Hypoechoic cervical mass, sometimes with internal septa ● Fluid–fluid levels may be found in hemorrhagic cysts.

▶ **CT findings**
Multilocular hypodense mass with enhancing fibrous septa ● Some hygromas are hyperdense due to intracystic hemorrhage ● Most important modality for investigating bony infiltration.

▶ **MRI findings**
Hyperintense on T2-weighted images, hypo- to isointense on T1-weighted images (lighter than muscle, darker than fat) ● Areas with high T1-weighted signal intensity are hemorrhagic cysts ● Septa enhance on T1-weighted images after gadolinium administration.

▶ **Pathognomonic findings**
Uni- or multilocular cystic mass ● Usually arises from the posterior cervical triangle and grows anteriorly ● Lesion grows by expansion but may also infiltrate muscles or vessels.

Clinical Aspects

▶ **Typical presentation**
Slowly enlarging mass ● Growth rate accelerated by intralesional hemorrhage or infection ● Small hygromas are asymptomatic ● Extensive cervical hygromas may cause signs of respiratory insufficiency, dysphagia, and/or facial paralysis ● Chylothorax and chylopericardium are rare.

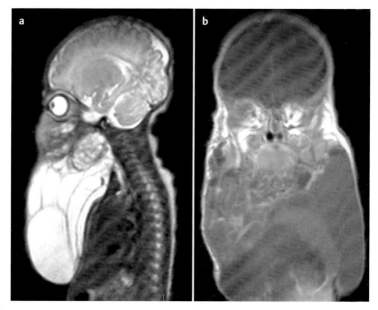

Fig. 9.11 a, b Sagittal STIR image (**a**) shows a large, septated, hyperintense submandibular mass draped over the front of the chest. Postgadolinium T1-weighted image (**b**) shows an inhomogeneous but predominantly hypointense mass with a hemorrhagic area and enhancing septa.

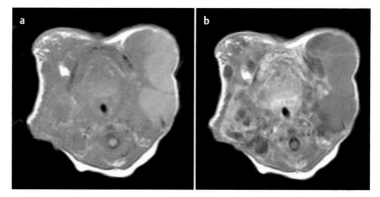

Fig. 9.12 a, b Axial T1-weighted images demonstrate large and small cysts of varying signal intensity due to intralesional hemorrhage (**a**) and interspersed enhancing connective tissue and septa following gadolinium administration (**b**).

Soft Tissues of the Neck

▶ **Treatment options**

Intrauterine masses require cesarean section to avoid fetal neck and airway trauma during delivery ● Primary treatment is tumor resection ● Only a subtotal resection can be done in many cases due to infiltration of soft-tissue and vascular structures ● *Alternative or adjunctive treatment options:* Laser therapy; sclerotherapy with 50% glucose, ethanol, hypertonic saline, or OK-432 (streptococcal preparation treated with benzylpenicillin).

▶ **Course and prognosis**

Good chance for a cure with complete resection ● Frequent recurrence after subtotal resection, especially with infiltration of the larynx, pharynx, floor of the mouth, or tongue ● Lower recurrence rate after OK-432 therapy.

▶ **What does the clinician want to know?**

Tumor extent ● Infiltration of organs and vessels.

Differential Diagnosis

Neck cysts (thyroglossal duct cyst, branchial cleft cyst)	– Noninfiltrating, unilocular, monocystic mass at a typical location (thyroglossal duct cyst: abutting the hyoid bone; branchial cleft cyst: anteromedial to vascular sheath)
Hemangioma	– No fluid–fluid level – Noninfiltrating
Teratoma, dermoid cyst	– Mixed cystic/solid tumor composed of various tissues (cartilage, teeth, muscle, hairs)
Cervical abscess	– Thick, enhancing septa around a liquid center with a perifocal reaction in surrounding tissues

Tips and Pitfalls

Infiltrative growth often raises false suspicion of a malignancy ● Infiltration of adjacent structures may be difficult to evaluate in very small children due to resolution limits.

Selected References

Koeller KK et al. Congenital cystic masses of the neck: Radiologic-pathologic correlation. Radiographics 1999; 19: 121–146

Trauffler PM et al. The natural history of euploid pregnacies with first-trimester cystic hygromas. Am J Obstetrics & Gynecology 1994; 170: 1279–1284

Yuh WT et al. Magnetic resonance imaging of pediatric head and neck cystic hygromas. Ann Otology, Rhinology & Laryngology 1991; 100: 737–742

Definition

▶ **Epidemiology**

Most common benign tumor in children ● Present in 2% of all children and 15% of all premature infants ● 60% in the head and neck region ● Accounts for 7% of all benign head and neck tumors ● More common in males (4:1).

▶ **Etiology, pathophysiology, pathogenesis**

Benign vascular tumor in children ● Often regresses spontaneously ● Usually cutaneous ● Endothelial cell proliferation may continue for 5–6 months after birth (proliferative phase) ● Hemangioma completely regresses by 4 years of age in 50% of cases and by 6 years in 70% (involution phase) ● Involution is sometimes incomplete, leaving residual changes ● Similar lesions in adults are called vascular malformations and do not regress.

Imaging Signs

▶ **Modality of choice**

MRI.

▶ **MRI findings**

Well-delineated lobular lesion ● Cutaneous or subcutaneous, sometimes intramuscular ● Iso- to hyperintense on T1-weighted images ● High T2-weighted signal intensity ● May contain linear or punctate foci of low signal intensity (flow voids in large vessels) ● Enhancement after gadolinium administration may be faint or intense, depending on vascularity, and may show early washout ● Possible deformation or hypertrophy of bony structures ● Bone infiltration is extremely rare.

▶ **Pathognomonic findings**

Sharply circumscribed lesion with high T2-weighted signal intensity showing immediate, intense, homogeneous enhancement after gadolinium administration.

Clinical Aspects

▶ **Typical presentation**

Characteristic clinical appearance of cutaneous hemangioma in an infant ● 96% are visible by age 5 months ● 80% are unilocular ● Subcutaneous or muscular hemangiomas may appear as a bluish soft-tissue swelling.

▶ **Treatment options**

Depend on the age of the child and the size, depth, and location of the tumor:
- Wait-and-see is justified for small lesions and in young children.
- < 2 mm deep, < 1.5 cm in diameter: Cryotherapy and dye laser.
- < 2 mm deep, located in the face: Nd:YAG laser.
- > 2 mm deep and > 1.5 cm in diameter, located in the eyelid: Surgical excision.
- Only very large lesions require cortisone and interferon therapy.

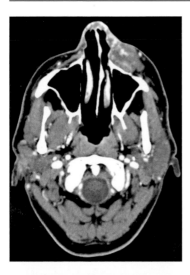

Fig. 9.13 Hemangioma of the left cheek. Postcontrast CT shows an inhomogeneous vascularized tumor located in the subcutaneous fat and extending to skin level with involvement of the left nostril.

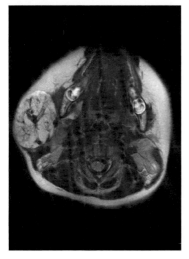

Fig. 9.14 Hemangioma in the right parotid compartment of a 1-year-old child. Plain T2-weighted MR image demonstrates a well-circumscribed, hyperintense tumor with a conspicuous mass effect. Vessels within the tumor appear as flow voids on the T2-weighted image. The ipsilateral parotid gland is displaced inferiorly.

▸ **Course and prognosis**
Good prognosis ● Spontaneous regression ● Residua in the form of pigmentary changes, scars, redundant skin, and ulcerations (40–50%) ● Possible association with intracranial and parenchymal malformations ● Complications (20–30% mortality): Kasabach–Merritt syndrome, compression of vital structures, bleeding, ulceration.

Differential Diagnosis

Vascular malformations	– Adults
	– Venous malformations: phleboliths
Lymphangioma	– Rarely cutaneous
	– No enhancement after contrast administration
Cystic hygroma	– Cystic structure
	– Fluid–fluid level
Neoplasms	– Diffuse, inhomogeneous enhancement, may contain necrotic areas
	– Invasive growth and ill-defined margins

Tips and Pitfalls

Hemangioma may be misdiagnosed as a malignant tumor.

Selected References

Chooi WK, Woodhouse N, Coley SC, Griffiths PD. Pediatric head and neck lesions: assessment of vascularity by MR digital subtraction angiography. AJNR Am J Neuroradiol 2004; 25(7): 1251–1255

Ernemann U, Hoffmann J, Gronewaller E, Breuninger H, Rebmann H, Adam C, Reinert S. Hämangiome und vaskuläre Malformationen im Kopf- und Halsbereich. Radiologe 2003; 43(11): 958–966

Robertson RL, Robson CD, Barnes PD, Burrows PE. Head and neck vascular anomalies of childhood. Neuroimaging Clin N Am 1999; 9(1): 115–132

Definition

▶ **Epidemiology**
Prevalence of primary hyperparathyroidism (Western population): 0.001–0.002% • 80% caused by solitary parathyroid adenoma • 15–20% by parathyroid hyperplasia • 0.05% by multiple adenomas and carcinomas of the parathyroid gland • More common in females (3:1) • Often postmenopausal in women.

▶ **Etiology, pathophysiology, pathogenesis**
Benign hyperplasia of the parathyroid gland with excessive parathormone secretion • Solitary in 85% of cases • Some cases have unknown etiology, some are genetic • Familial causes (FHH, MEN 1, MEN 2A) should be excluded in children and adolescents • Parathyroid adenoma is the leading cause of hypercalcemia.

Imaging Signs

▶ **Modality of choice**
MRI • Image fusion of MRI with ^{99m}Tc-MIBI SPECT • Sonography.

▶ **CT findings**
Frequent inhomogeneous (central hypodense) arterial enhancement and homogeneous venous enhancement.

▶ **MRI findings**
Rounded masses sometimes permeated by fibrotic or hemorrhagic changes • *Sites of occurrence:* preesophageal, paraesophageal, juxtathyroid, retrothyroid, rarely intrathyroid or ectopic location in cervical soft tissues or mediastinum • Parathyroid adenomas and hyperplasia show high T2-weighted signal intensity and increased T1-weighted signal intensity after gadolinium administration • Diagnosis is often difficult postoperatively and in patients with a goiter • MRI has 62–94% sensitivity in the detection of parathyroid adenomas, 54–75% in the detection of hyperplasia.

▶ **Selected normal values**
Normal parathyroid gland: 3–10 mm × 2–6 mm × 2–4 mm.
Parathyroid adenoma: 6–30 mm × 5–15 mm × 3–8 mm.

▶ **Pathognomonic findings**
Signal characteristics are virtually specific for lesions at typical sites showing a typical size and enhancement pattern.

Clinical Aspects

▶ **Typical presentation**
Many patients present with hypercalcemia, renal stones, and possible bone fractures • Hard nodules, 2–3 mm in size, are palpable in rare cases • *Laboratory tests:* Serum calcium, parathormone, 24-hour urine.

▶ **Treatment options**
Open or minimally invasive surgical removal on one or both sides • *Complications:* Recurrent laryngeal nerve palsy (1–3%), vascular injury, persistence of hypersecretory parathyroid tissue.

Fig. 9.15 Parathyroid adenoma at a right retrothyroid location. Plain T2-weighted MR image. The tumor appears as a rounded mass with high T2-weighted signal intensity (arrow).

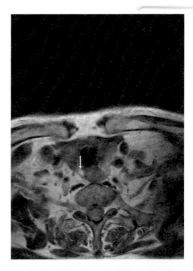

Fig. 9.16 a, b Postcontrast axial CT (**a**) of a left retrothyroid adenoma of the parathyroid gland (arrow) located adjacent to the esophagus. The tumor appears slightly hypodense to the thyroid tissue. On plain axial CT (**b**) the adenoma is hyperdense to the blood vessels (arrow).

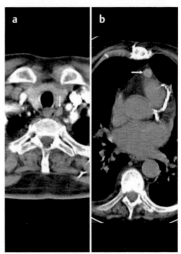

▶ **Course and prognosis**

98% cure rate with unilateral or bilateral parathyroidectomy ● Symptoms persist in rare cases ● Minimally invasive removal is as effective as open surgery and has lower complication rates.

Differential Diagnosis

Parathyroid carcinoma	– Often larger
	– Locally invasive growth
	– Lymph node metastases
Lymphadenopathy (malignant, granulomatous or inflammatory)	– Often multiple
	– Diffuse enhancement after contrast administration
	– Possible central necrosis
	– No hilum
	– Inflammatory perifocal reaction
Hamartoma, lipoadenoma	– Contain fatty tissue (high T1-weighted signal intensity)
	– Fibrotic

Tips and Pitfalls

Small adenomas may be missed if scintigraphy is omitted ● Limiting the field of view to the head and neck region may cause ectopic adenomas to be missed.

Selected References

Delorme S, Hoffner S. Diagnostik des Hyperparathyreodismus. Radiologe 2003; 43(4): 275–283

Ruf J, Hänninen L, Steinmüller Th, Rohlfing T, Bertram H et al. Präoperative Lokalisations-diagnostik von Nebenschilddrüsen: Nutzen der MRT, Szintigraphie und Bildfusion. Nuklearmedizin 2004; 43: 85–90

Sekiyama K, Akakura K, Mikami K, Mizoguchi K, Tobe T, Nakano K, Numata T, Konno A, Ito H. Usefulness of diagnostic imaging in primary hyperparathyroidism. Int J Urol 2003; 10(1): 7–11

Weber AL, Randolph G, Aksoy FG. The thyroid and parathyroid glands. CT and MR imaging and correlation with pathology and clinical findings. Radiol Clin North Am 2000; 38(5): 1105–1129

Soft Tissues of the Neck

Definition

▶ **Epidemiology**
Incidence varies greatly by geography, being higher in areas that are inland and far from the sea ● 740 million people are affected worldwide (13% endemic) ● Incidence increases with age ● Male-to-female ratio: 1:2–4.5 ● 95% of goiters are benign, 5% are malignant.

▶ **Etiology, pathophysiology, pathogenesis**
Enlargement of the thyroid gland, usually due to nodular hyperplasia ● Iodine deficiency is the most frequent causal factor (minimum iodine requirement: 1 μg/kg body weigth/day) ● Reduced iodine intake decreases growth inhibition ● *Genetic component:* Goiter is more prevalent in children with affected parents ● Cases are classified functionally as euthyroid or hyperthyroid.

Imaging Signs

▶ **Modality of choice**
Sonography ● Then scintigraphy ($^{99\,m}$Tc pertechnate) ● MRI and CT are very useful for investigating retrosternal and intrathoracic extension.

▶ **CT findings**
Calcifications (amorphous, eggshell) are present in 90% of cases ● Hemorrhagic and hypodense colloidal areas ● CT is particularly useful for evaluating intrathoracic extension.

▶ **MRI findings**
MRI usually shows an enlarged thyroid gland with inhomogeneous T1- and T2-weighted signal characteristics (colloids, blood) ● The organ capsule is intact and well delineated ● Bilateral displacement of the neurovascular sheath ● Possible tracheal compression ● May extend inferiorly to the level of the aortic arch ● Extrathyroid extension is present in 44% of cases, is often retrosternal.

▶ **Sonographic findings**
Enlarged thyroid gland with an intact capsule ● Nonhomogeneous internal echo pattern ● Sharply circumscribed cystic (hypoechoic) and solid (often hyperechoic) nodules, usually hypovascular (color duplex sonography) ● "Eggshell" calcifications.

▶ **Selected normal values**
Dimensions of thyroid gland: craniocaudal 3.5–6 cm, transverse 1.5–2 cm, sagittal 1–2 cm.

▶ **Pathognomonic findings**
Enlarged, inhomogeneously enhancing thyroid gland with smooth margins and multiple dense (hyperplasia), cystic (degeneration) and calcified areas. A malignant goiter cannot be diagnosed from MR and CT images alone.

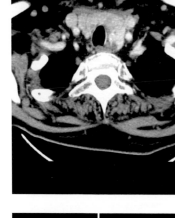

Fig. 9.17 Multinodular goiter. Postcontrast CT scan shows inhomogeneous thyroid tissue with multiple hypodense areas and a small eggshell calcification in the left thyroid lobe. The patient had normal TSH and normal peripheral thyroid hormone levels.

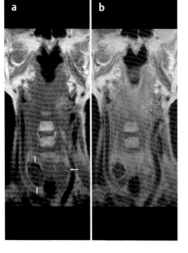

Fig. 9.18 a, b T1-weighted MR image before (**a**) and after gadolinium administration (**b**). Multinodular goiter. The precontrast image (**a**) shows inhomogeneous thyroid tissue with some very hypointense areas (mostly calcifications, vertical lines). Areas of intermediate SI are accompanied by slightly hyperintense areas (arrow). The postcontrast image (**b**) shows no enhancement of areas with regressive changes.

Clinical Aspects

▶ **Typical presentation**

Often an incidental finding ● Higher incidence in iodine-deficient geographic regions.

WHO classification:

– Grade 0: No goiter.
– Grade I a: Palpable, not visible.
– Grade I b: Visible only with the head tilted back.
– Grade II: Visible with the head in a normal position.
– Grade III: Plainly visible.

Possible complications of grade III goiter: 55% airway narrowing, 15% hoarseness, 10% dysphagia, 10% vena cava compression ● Laboratory values often normal (TSH, fT3, fT4) ● Occasional Graves' disease with "Merseburg triad" of tachycardia, goiter, and exophthalmos (in 40–60%).

▶ **Treatment options**

Prophylaxis (e.g., with iodized salt) ● Mild goiter treatable with iodide and levothyroxine (< 30% volume reduction) ● Subtotal to total thyroidectomy for grade III goiters (and grade II goiters unresponsive to conservative treatment), hyperthyroidism, or malignant goiter ● If thyroidectomy is contraindicated, an alternative is radioiodine therapy (30% volume reduction).

▶ **Course and prognosis**

Surgery plus radioiodine therapy is curative ● Thyroidectomy should be followed by hormone replacement therapy ● Complications of first operation: < 3% rate of permanent recurrent laryngeal nerve palsy (up to 20% in reoperations), < 1% (< 5%) hypocalcemia, < 4% (4%) bleeding, < 2% (< 2%) infection, and 0% (< 1%) mortality.

Differential Diagnosis

Thyroid carcinoma, undifferentiated (medullary and anaplastic)	– More rapid and invasive growth, breaches thyroid capsule – Lymph node metastases – Encases neurovascular sheath
Thyroid carcinoma, differentiated (papillary and follicular)	– Faster growing, may transgress the capsule – Not positively distinguishable from goiter by MRI and CT
Follicular thyroid adenoma	– Solitary, noninvasive intrathyroid focus – Solid, enhancing – Differentiation very difficult
Non-Hodgkin lymphoma	– Rarely necrotic or calcified – Relatively rapid growth – Uniformly hypointense or hypodense to normal thyroid tissue
Hemorrhagic colloid cyst	– Intrathyroid mass with cystic boundaries – Normal thyroid tissue

Tips and Pitfalls

Benign goiters have a bizarre imaging appearance that can mimic malignancy.

Selected References

Czerny C, Hormann M, Kurtaran A, Niederle B. Imaging of diseases of the thyroid gland in Austria. Wien Klin Wochenschr 2003; 115 Suppl 2: 71–74

Hegedüs L, Bonnema, SJ, Bennedbaek, F Management of Simple Nodular Goiter: Current Status and Future Perspectives 2003 Endocrine Reviews 24(1): 102–132

Weber AL, Randolph G, Aksoy FG. The thyroid and parathyroid glands. CT and MR imaging and correlation with pathology and clinical findings. Radiol Clin North Am 2000; 38(5): 1105–1129

Definition

▶ **Epidemiology**
More common in males (2:1) • 1% of all malignant tumors • 94% are differentiated carcinomas (peak incidence at 45–55 years): 85% papillary, 15% follicular • 6% are undifferentiated carcinoma: 5% medullary (30 years), 1% anaplastic (70 years) • Special form of follicular carcinoma: Oncocytic carcinoma (more aggressive in 20%).

▶ **Etiology, pathophysiology, pathogenesis**
Malignant tumor arising from thyroid tissue • Association with goiter (20–30%) and MEN 2 • *Papillary carcinoma:* Induced by ionizing radiation, 5–10% are hereditary • *Anaplastic carcinoma:* Most are completely dedifferentiated.

Imaging Signs

▶ **Modality of choice**
Sonography, supplemented if necessary by MRI.

▶ **CT findings**
Mixed hyper- and hypodense pattern • Anaplastic carcinoma is associated with necrosis in 75% of cases, calcifications in 60%, lymph node metastasis in 40%, and distant metastasis in 25% • *Follicular carcinoma:* Lymph node metastasis in 30%, distant metastasis in 22% at time of diagnosis • *Oncocytic carcinoma:* Lymph node metastasis in 21%, distant metastasis in 33% at time of diagnosis.

▶ **MRI findings**
Mixed high and low signal intensity on T1- and T2-weighted images • Plain imaging is important because thyroglobulin and intralesional hemorrhage are hyperintense on plain images but are masked by gadolinium administration.

▶ **Sonographic findings**
Ten percent are bilateral • Invasive growth • Frequent irregular margins • Transcapsular growth indicates malignancy • Infiltration of the trachea, esophagus, and recurrent laryngeal nerve.

▶ **Selected normal values**
Normal dimensions of the thyroid gland: Craniocaudal 3.5–6 cm, transverse 1.5–2 cm, sagittal 1–2 cm.

▶ **Pathognomonic findings**
Different types cannot be distinguished by CT and MRI.

Clinical Aspects

▶ **Typical presentation**
Fast-growing nodule in the thyroid gland • Possible visible neck swelling • Dysphagia, dyspnea, or superior vena cava compression • Frequent elevation of calcitonin and CEA • Anaplastic carcinoma often goes undetected until stage T4 • No iodine uptake after pentagastrin stimulation.

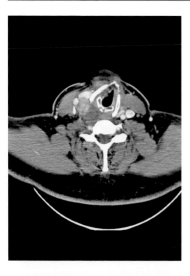

Fig. 9.19 Postcontrast CT scan of thyroid carcinoma at the level of the thyroid cartilage on the right side. The tumor has a complex structure consisting of hypodense necrotic areas, hyperdense hemorrhagic areas, and areas showing intense enhancement after contrast administration. The carcinoma has displaced the larynx and neurovascular sheath anteriorly. A cutaneous defect is noted anterior to the tumor.

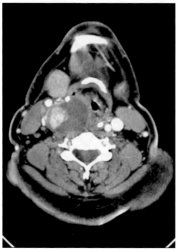

Fig. 9.20 Postcontrast CT (same patient as in Fig. 9.**19**) shows extensive vertical, cephalad extension of the thyroid carcinoma. The tumor contains a combination of hypodense cystic areas, hyperdense hemorrhagic areas, and areas of intense enhancement. A large, hyperdense lymph node metastasis is visible in the right submandibular area directly anterior to the tumor.

▶ **Treatment options**

Thyroidectomy with central lymphadenectomy, recurrent laryngeal nerve identification, and preservation of at least one parathyroid gland • Radioiodine therapy.

▶ **Course and prognosis**

The course and prognosis vary considerably depending on the histologic tumor type:

- Papillary and follicular: Postoperative radioiodine therapy for 4 weeks, levothyroxine for life.
- Anaplastic: Average survival time 10 months.
- Medullary: 10-year survival rate of 80%.
- Complication rate same as goiter (p. 228).

Differential Diagnosis

Follicular thyroid adenoma	– Solitary, noninvasive intrathyroid focus
	– Solid, enhancing
	– Differentiation very difficult
Nodular or diffuse goiter	– Noninvasive, does not breach the capsule
	– Gradual enlargement
Non-Hodgkin lymphoma	– Relatively homogeneous appearance, rarely shows necrosis
	– No calcifications or intralesional hemorrhage
Hemorrhagic colloid cyst	– Intrathyroid mass with cystic boundaries
	– Normal thyroid tissue

Tips and Pitfalls

Caution: The use of iodinated contrast medium delays radioiodine therapy.

Selected References

Casella C, Fusco M. Thyroid cancer. Epidemiol Prev 2004; 28(2 Suppl): 88–91

Gross ND, Weissman JL, Talbot JM, Andersen PE, Wax MK, Cohen JI. MRI detection of cervical metastasis from differentiated thyroid carcinoma. Laryngoscope 2001; 111(11 Pt 1): 1905–1909

Takashima S, Matsushita T, Takayama F, Kadoya M, Fujimori M, Kobayashi T. Prognostic significance of magnetic resonance findings in advanced papillary thyroid cancer. Thyroid 2001; 11(12): 1153–1159

Definition

Posttherapeutic cervical changes following the treatment of head and neck tumors.

▶ **Epidemiology**
Found routinely in oncologic patients following radiation to the neck, radical neck dissection, modified neck dissection, or selective neck dissection.

▶ **Etiology, pathophysiology, pathogenesis**
Radiation-induced changes: Depend on radiation type, dose, and portal. Initial change is edema due to endothelial damage (blood vessels and lymphatics), followed later by fibrosis and atrophy.
Postoperative changes:
– Radical neck dissection: Level I–V lymphadenectomy, jugular vein, CN XI, sternocleidomastoid muscle.
– Modified neck dissection: Preserves one or more functional structures.
– Selective neck dissection: Selective lymphadenectomy at levels I–V.

Imaging Signs

▶ **Modality of choice**
MRI, CT.

▶ **CT findings**
Radiation-induced changes: Decreased density and increased volume (edema) of the skin, subcutaneous tissue, epiglottis, retro- and parapharyngeal space, laryngeal soft tissues (rarely cartilage), and salivary glands. Later changes: atrophy of salivary glands (chiefly the parotid) • Bone-marrow edema (mandible, cervical spine), fatty degeneration, osteonecrosis.
Postoperative changes: Depend on the type of operation (selective neck dissection, modified neck dissection, radical neck dissection). Ipsilateral absence of level I–V lymph nodes, jugular vein, CN XI, sternocleidomastoid muscle, immediate postoperative edema, later scar formation and atrophy.

▶ **MRI findings**
Radiation-induced changes: Swelling with high T2-weighted and low T2-weighted signal intensity • Increased T1-weighted signal intensity after gadolinium administration • Increased T2-weighted signal intensity in mastoid cells with no enhancement after gadolinium administration in T1-weighted image • Bone marrow acquires high T1-weighted signal intensity and intermediate T2-weighted signal intensity due to fatty degeneration • Inflammatory fibrous reaction shows increased signal intensity in the tumor bed on T2-weighted images and after gadolinium administration.
Postoperative changes: See CT Findings above.

▶ **Pathognomonic findings**
Radiation-induced changes: Cervical edema (usually symmetrical), skin thickening, fatty bone-marrow degeneration, and salivary gland atrophy.
Postoperative changes: Unilateral absence of cervical lymph nodes or functional structures with asymmetry of cervical soft tissues.

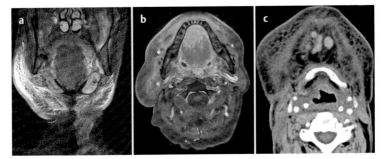

Fig. 9.21 a–c Coronal STIR sequence (**a**) shows predominantly right-sided edema with increased signal intensity in the subcutaneous and parapharyngeal tissues and submandibular glands. Axial T1-weighted image (**b**) after gadolinium administration (same patient as in **a**) shows enhancement of the subcutaneous tissue, oropharynx, tongue, parapharyngeal space, and right parotid gland. **c** Marked submandibular edema. Note the submental lymph nodes.

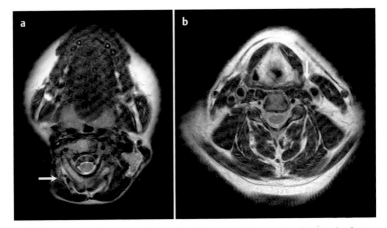

Fig. 9.22 a, b Unenhanced axial T2-weighted images. **a** Asymmetry of cervical soft tissues following a radical neck dissection on the right side that included removal of the sternocleidomastoid muscle, jugular vein, CN XI, and cervical lymph nodes. There is partial atrophy of the right semispinalis capitis (arrow), which is innervated by C4–T6 spinal nerves. **b** Image after a modified neck dissection shows absence of the left jugular vein. Cervical fatty tissue was spared, and small lymph nodes are visible on the left side (arrow).

Clinical Aspects

▶ **Typical presentation**
Radiation-induced changes:
  – Early changes: Mucositis, ageusia, hyposalivation.
  – Late sequelae: Hyposalivation, caries, periodontitis, trismus, osteoradionecrosis, dysphagia, carotid stenosis, stroke.
Postoperative changes: Asymmetry of cervical soft tissues, trapezius atrophy, shoulder pain, limited shoulder abduction (CN XI lesion).

▶ **Treatment options**
Before radiotherapy: Extraction of critical teeth, antibiotics, hyperbaric oxygen therapy (HBO), debridement (osteoradionecrotic foci in the mandible).
Radiation-induced changes: Oral hygiene, antibiotics, fluorine (mucositis, caries, periodontitis), artificial saliva, copious fluids, sialogogue (hyposalivation).
Postoperative changes: Flap reconstruction, physical therapy, Eden–Lange reconstruction of shoulder muscles.

▶ **Course and prognosis**
Radiation-induced changes: Edema should regress by 6–12 months after treatment ● Doses ≥ 60 Gy usually cause permanent salivary gland atrophy with hyposalivation ● Life-long problems with dental caries.
Postoperative changes: Regional lymph node recurrence rate is 2 % for preoperative stage pN0, 26 % for multiple nodal and extranodal involvement, and 7 % after postoperative radiation to the neck ● Risk of osteoradionecrosis.

▶ **What does the clinician want to know?**
Correlation between anatomic changes and symptoms ● Residual tumor, recurrence, or lymph node recurrence? Osteoradionecrosis? Muscular atrophy?

Differential Diagnosis

Residual tumor or recurrence	– Asymmetrical mass with high T2-weighted signal intensity, low T1-weighted signal intensity, and enhancement after gadolinium administration

Tips and Pitfalls

Certain bilateral tumors may be indistinguishable from edema ● Except for tumor growth, there is no imaging criterion for distinguishing residual tumor from a radiation-induced inflammatory reaction in the tumor bed ● Status after selective neck dissection or modified neck dissection may be missed on images.

Selected References

Nömayr A et al. MRI appearance of radiation-induced changes of normal cervical tissues. Eur Radiol 2001; 11: 1807–1817

Hudgins PA et al. Selective neck dissection: CT and MR imaging findings. AJNR Am J Neuroradiol 2005; 26: 1174–1177

Anatomy

▶ **Location**

Anatomically, the neck is drained by 10 groups of lymph nodes that communicate with one another (see table). The AJCC classification of the cervical lymph nodes into seven levels is more important for clinical purposes (p. 249).

▶ **Shape**

Normal lymph nodes have an oval shape ● The long axis is parallel to the major blood vessels ● In lymph nodes with a longitudinal diameter of 1–2 cm, the ratio of the longitudinal to transverse diameter (L/T ratio) is ≥ 2.

Lymph node group	Normal size	Regions drained
Occipital	Not definable by CT or MRI	Occipital scalp
Postauricular	Not definable by CT or MRI	Parietal scalp
Parotid	< 6 mm	Frontal and parietal scalp, orbit, parotid gland
Submandibular	< 10 mm	Orbit, tongue, mouth, submandibular gland, anterior nose
Facial	Not definable by CT or MRI	Orbit, anterior nose
Submental	< 10 mm	Oral cavity, tongue
Sublingual	Not definable by CT or MRI	Floor of the mouth, tongue
Retropharyngeal	< 6 mm	Paranasal sinuses, nasopharynx, oropharynx, posterior nose, cervical esophagus
Anterior cervical	Not definable by CT or MRI	Larynx, thyroid gland, cervical esophagus
Lateral cervical		
● Superficial cervical	Not definable by CT or MRI	Skin of the neck
● Deep cervical		
– Cranial jugular nodes	< 15 mm	All regions
– Medial jugular nodes	< 10 mm	All regions
– Caudal jugular nodes	< 10 mm	All regions

CT Anatomy

▶ **Examination technique**
Contrast-enhanced CT ● Slice thickness ≤ 3 mm ● Sagittal reformatting is advised.

▶ **Size and shape**
Often only the transverse diameter is measured in axial scans ● Normal transverse diameter is ≤ 10 mm ● Normal maximum longitudinal diameter in reformatted spiral images is 10–15 mm ● Reniform configuration is common due to central fatty infiltration of the medulla (hypodense) in the setting of fibrolipomatous degeneration (hilar fat sign).

▶ **Contrast characteristics**
Moderate homogeneous enhancement.

MRI

▶ **Examination technique**
- Phased-array coil.
- *Nonenhanced*: Axial and coronal T2-weighted images, supplemented if necessary by sagittal T1-weighted images or coronal STIR images.
- *With gadolinium*: Axial T1-weighted images with fat suppression, supplemented if necessary by sagittal or coronal images.
- *With USPIO*: Axial and coronal T1-weighted images, coronal T2-weighted images with fat suppression.

▶ **Size and shape**
Same as CT ● Usual maximum size is in the range of 10–15 mm.

▶ **Signal characteristics**
Usually isointense to muscle on T1-weighted images ● Fatty infiltration of medulla in fibrolipomatous degeneration shows high T1-weighted signal intensity ● Hyperintense to muscle on T2-weighted images, iso- or hypointense to fat ● Lymph nodes are markedly hyperintense to their generally hypointense surroundings in fat-suppressed T2-weighted and STIR images.

▶ **Contrast characteristics**
Gadolinium: Homogeneous enhancement after gadolinium administration ● Well-delineated high signal intensity on fat-suppressed T1-weighted images.
USPIO: Low, homogeneous T2-weighted signal 24 hours after USPIO administration due to uniform iron uptake ● Narrow hyperintense rim may be seen.

Sonography

▶ **Examination technique**
High-frequency transducer (5–10 MHz) ● Lymph nodes are individually defined and evaluated in their longitudinal and transverse dimensions ● Intranodal vessels can be assessed by color duplex sonography ● The degree and pattern of vascularity are evaluated ● Sample volume is positioned in the largest vessel to record a Doppler spectrum.

▶ **Size and shape**

Normally smaller than 15 mm ● Oblong shape ● Sonography is the best modality for defining longitudinal and transverse nodal diameters and calculating the ratios ● L/T ratio ≥ 2 is normal for lymph nodes with a diameter > 10 mm ● The L/T ratio is not a reliable criterion for lymph nodes smaller than 10 mm (measurement error).

▶ **Echo characteristics**

Hypoechoic cortex with high-amplitude hilar echoes ● Sharply defined margins ● Color duplex may show no detectable vascularity or homogeneous vascularity throughout the lymph node.

Normal Findings in Children

▶ **Sonographic findings**

Fine, homogeneous echo texture with moderate echogenicity ● Normally indistinguishable from surrounding connective tissue.

▶ **MRI findings**

Signal characteristics identical to cervical lymph nodes in adults: Isointense to muscle on T1-weighted images and hyperintense to muscle on T2-weighted images.

Definition

▶ **Epidemiology**
Common condition in children ● 50% occur by 5 years of age, 90% by age 10 ●
Less common in adults.

▶ **Etiology, pathophysiology, pathogenesis**
Inflammatory lymphadenopathy of the cervical soft tissues.
Acute cervical lymphadenitis: Main causative organisms are streptococci and
staphylococci (40–80%), and anaerobes ● Usually precipitated by a focal inflammation of the nose, mouth, ears, pharynx, or skin.
Subacute or chronic lymphadenitis: Caused by tuberculosis, atypical mycobacteriosis, toxoplasmosis, or cat-scratch disease ● Rare variants of uncertain etiology
are most prevalent in Asia: Kikuchi–Fujimoto disease (histiocytic necrotizing
lymphadenitis).

Imaging Signs

▶ **Modality of choice**
Sonography ● Contrast-enhanced CT.

▶ **Sonographic findings**
Acute lymphadenitis: Affected nodes are elongated (L/T ratio >>2) ● Cortex is
slightly hypoechoic ● Central hilar echo ● Sharp outer margins ● Hypervascularity with central hilar vessel.
Chronic lymphadenitis: Same as acute lymphadenitis, but without detectable vascularity.

▶ **CT findings**
Enlarged, oval lymph nodes in the region draining the focal infection ● Usually
shows homogeneous enhancement after contrast administration ● Central cavitation creates a hypodense, nonenhancing center with peripheral rim enhancement ● Possible imbibition of surrounding fat and skin thickening ● Usually unilateral ● Central cavitation is common in nontuberculous mycobacterial infection.

▶ **MRI findings**
Affected lymph nodes show low T1-weighted and high T2-weighted signal intensity ● Homogeneous enhancement after gadolinium administration ● Central cavitation has low signal intensity on postgadolinium T1-weighted images.

▶ **Pathognomonic findings**
Enlarged, elongated lymph nodes with L/T ratio >>2 ● Homogeneous enhancement after contrast administration ● Possible central cavitation ● Typically unilateral in acute bacterial infections ● Density of surrounding fat is often increased ● Nontuberculous mycobacterial lymphadenitis often associated with
salivary gland infiltration in the submandibular region or parotid compartment.

Fig. 10.1 Cervical lymphadenitis. Axial CT showing an enlarged lymph node with central cavitation. The margins are indistinct and there is rim enhancement posterior to the left internal jugular vein and medial to the sternocleidomastoid muscle.

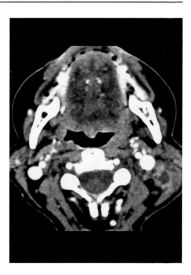

Clinical Aspects

▶ **Typical presentation**

Acute lymphadenitis: The swelling most commonly involves the upper and central anterior cervical soft tissues and submandibular region • Typically unilateral • Neck pain • Limited neck movement • Prior history of upper respiratory or dental infection • Lymph nodes swollen and tender on palpation.

Chronic lymphadenitis: More prolonged and severe lymph node swelling that does not regress over time • No acute exacerbation • Subfebrile temperatures only • Generally mild symptoms.

Kikuchi–Fujimoto disease: Predominantly affects females, 10–30 years of age • Leukopenia • 50% present with low-grade fever, lethargy, and diarrhea • Possible nausea and vomiting • Bilateral lymph node enlargement in 20% of cases.

▶ **Treatment options**

Acute lymphadenitis: Parenteral antibiotics (penicillin, second and third generation cephalosporins) • Incision and drainage of abscess • Treatment of underlying disease.

Chronic lymphadenitis: Treatment of underlying disease (e.g., antituberculous drugs, pyrimethamine for toxoplasmosis) • Combination chemotherapy for atypical mycobacteriosis • Local lymphadenectomy, possibly with excision of affected salivary glands • Amelioration of immune status.

Kikuchi–Fujimoto disease: Usually self-limiting.

▶ **Course and prognosis**

Acute lymphadenitis: Prompt, complete resolution with antibiotic therapy • Important to treat the portal of entry (e.g., tooth extraction).

Chronic lymphadenitis: Depends on causative organism ● Atypical mycobacteriosis has a good prognosis after complete surgical excision.

Kikuchi–Fujimoto disease: Usually resolves spontaneously in 8–10 months.

▶ **What does the clinician want to know?**
Affected groups of lymph nodes ● Lymph node size ● Perifocal reaction ● Cavitation ● Changes in neighboring structures.

Differential Diagnosis

Reactive lymphadenopathy	– Most common in viral infections of the upper respiratory tract
	– Usually painless, noncavitating lymph node enlargement
Infectious mononucleosis	– Generalized swollen lymph nodes with fever and sore throat
	– Hepatosplenomegaly
Lymphoma, metastases	– Painless lymph node swelling
	– Possible cavitation
	– Systemic manifestations (fever, night sweats, weight loss)

Tips and Pitfalls

Imaging features of lymphadenopathy may be mistaken for lymphoma or metastasis ● Always correlate with clinical findings ● Look for a possible primary focus of infection.

Selected References

Cengiz AB et al. Acute neck infections in children. Turk J Pediatr 2004; 46: 153–158

Danielides Vet al. Diagnosis, Management and Surgical Treatment of Non-Tuberculous Mycobacterial Head and Neck Infection in Children. ORL 2002; 64: 284–289

Soon-Young K et al. CT Findings in Kikuchi Disease: Analysis of 69 cases. Am J Neuroradiol 2004; 25: 1099–1102

Definition

▶ **Epidemiology**
Incidence in western Europe: 5–20:100 000 per year • Male preponderance •
High-risk groups: AIDS patients, alcoholics, drug addicts, homeless, elderly • An
estimated 50 million people have multiresistant tuberculosis worldwide.

▶ **Etiology, pathophysiology, pathogenesis**
Factors that lower host resistance and increase the risk of tuberculosis include
malnutrition, diabetes mellitus, lymphoma, HIV, and silicosis • With an intact
immune system, only 5% of people infected with *Mycobacterium tuberculosis*
will contract the disease • 20% of AIDS patients develop tuberculosis • Cervical
tuberculosis is a postprimary disease caused by hematogenous spread in 90% of
cases (local manifestation of a systemic disease) • Primary orocervical infection
in 5% • Acid-fast bacilli (*M. tuberculosis* and *M. bovis*) are usually transmitted by
droplet infection.

Imaging Signs

▶ **Modality of choice**
Sonography • Contrast-enhanced CT.

▶ **Sonographic findings**
Enlarged lymph nodes • Echo-free to hypoechoic center • Lymph nodes tend to
form conglomerates in active tuberculosis • Calcifications produce high-amplitude echoes • Color duplex sonography shows displaced intranodal vessels.

▶ **CT findings**
Enlarged lymph nodes, often arranged in clusters • Central hypodensity due to
cavitation • Ring enhancement seen in 90% of acute cases (broader ring than
metastatic nodes: > 20% of diameter) • Chronic cases often develop flocculent
or homogeneous calcifications.

▶ **MRI findings**
Lymph node enlargement • Nonspecific signal characteristics • Cavitation
causes ring enhancement after gadolinium administration with central low T1-
weighted signal intensity and high T2-weighted signal intensity.

▶ **Pathognomonic findings**
Usually bilateral and/or multiple lymph node enlargement • Involved lymph nodes often located in posterior and inferior neck regions • Cavitation causes central low density on CT and ring enhancement after contrast administration.

Clinical Aspects

▶ **Typical presentation**
Usually has a subacute to chronic course • Moderately firm lymph node swel-
ling, often bilateral • Mild systemic manifestations • Subfebrile temperatures •
Night sweats • Weight loss • Little if any pain • Prone to cutaneous infiltration
and fistulation • There is often a history of unsuccessful antibiotic therapy •
Positive tuberculin skin test • Culture is the gold standard for diagnosis.

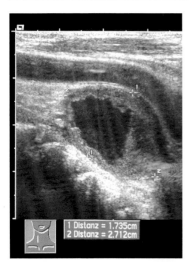

Fig. 10.2 Tuberculosis. Sonographic appearance of an enlarged, centrally hypoechoic cervical lymph node in a 15-year-old boy with HIV and tuberculosis.

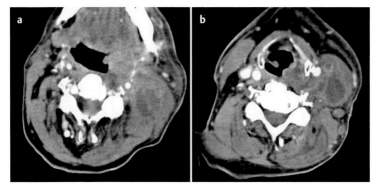

Fig. 10.3 a, b Axial CT shows a large, cavitating neck mass medial to the left sternocleidomastoid muscle (**a**). Lymph node with ill-defined margins, broad rim enhancement, and perifocal reaction accompanied by two adjacent cavitated nodes (**b**).

Lymph Nodes

▶ **Treatment options**

Primary conservative treatment: Triple tuberculostatic drug therapy (isoniazid, rifampicin, pyrazinamide) for 6–9 months ● *Adjuvant surgical treatment:* Only in patients with large, conglomerate nodal masses with central cavitation or fistulation.

▶ **Course and prognosis**

More than 90% of infections are clinically silent ● Treatment response depends on associated resistance-lowering diseases and early initiation of therapy.

▶ **What does the clinician want to know?**

Detection and localization of affected lymph nodes ● Cavitation ● Evidence of fistulation.

Differential Diagnosis

Nontuberculous myco-bacterial lymphadenitis	– Mainly affects small children – Usually unilateral – Usually affects only one group of lymph nodes – Predominantly affects submandibular or preauricular nodes – Systemic manifestations are rare
Sarcoidosis	– Firm, bilateral lymph node swelling – Frequent supraclavicular involvement – Usually associated with bihilar lymphadenopathy – Often resolves with formation of coarse calcifications
Lymphomas	– Generalized involvement common in NHL – Cavitation rare in Hodgkin disease

Tips and Pitfalls

Tuberculous cervical lymphadenopathy can be difficult to distinguish from abscess formation and cavitating tumor necrosis ● *Important:* Always consider tuberculosis in the differential diagnosis of cervical lymphadenopathy.

Selected References

Jäckel MC, Sattler B. Tuberkulöse und nichttuberkulöse mykobakterielle Erkrankungen der Halslymphknoten. HNO 2001; 49: 320–333

Reede DL, Bergeron RT. Cervical tuberculous adenitis: CT manifestations. Radiology 1985; 154: 701–704

Ying M et al. Accuracy of sonographic vascular features in differentiating different causes of cervical lymphadenopathy. Ultrasound Med Biol 2004; 30 (4): 441–447

Definition

▶ **Epidemiology**

Hodgkin disease, Hodgkin lymphoma (HL): Incidence 3:100 000 per year • More common in males (3:2 ratio) • Bimodal peak at approximately 30 and 60 years of age • Cervical involvement is most common.

Non-Hodgkin lymphoma (NHL): Incidence 5–10/100 000 per year • More common in males (1.5:1) • Most prevalent in older individuals • Incidence 1000 times higher in AIDS patients • *Affected cell line:* B-cell line in 80–85%, T-cell line in 15–20% • Second most common head and neck neoplasm (5%) • 50% nodal involvement, 10–20% extranodal involvement.

▶ **Etiology, pathophysiology, pathogenesis**

– *Hodgkin disease:* Etiology unknown • Association with Epstein–Barr virus.
– *NHL:* Association with Epstein–Barr and HTLV-1 viruses • Some cases show tumor-specific gene mutation.

▶ **Staging**

Ann Arbor classification:

– Stage I: Involvement of a single lymph node region • Localized involvement of a single extralymphatic organ.
– Stage II: Involvement of two or more lymph node regions on the same side of the diaphragm • Localized involvement of one extralymphatic organ. and/or regional lymph nodes and/or other lymph node regions on the same side of the diaphragm.
– Stage III: Involvement of lymph node regions on both sides of the diaphragm and/or localized involvement of one extralymphatic organ.
– Stage IV: Disseminated (multifocal) involvement of extralymphatic organs and/or regional lymph node involvement.

Imaging Signs

▶ **Modality of choice**

Sonography • Contrast-enhanced CT.

▶ **Sonographic findings**

Increase in size and number of lymph nodes • Usually display a spherical shape • Very low echogenicity • Frequent absence of hilar echo • Well-defined margins • Pronounced hypervascularity with arborizing intranodal vascular pattern on color duplex images • High intranodal resistance index (RI < 0.8).

▶ **CT findings**

Affected lymph nodes are isodense to muscle • Nodes tend to form conglomerates • Lymph nodes usually show homogeneous density • Nodes in Hodgkin disease may show central low density as sign of necrosis • Minimal enhancement after contrast administration • Rarely, intense enhancement is seen in NHL • Calcifications usually do not form until after therapy.

▶ **MRI findings**

Affected lymph nodes are isointense to muscle on T1-weighted images and hyperintense on T2-weighted and STIR images • Like CT, usually shows homoge-

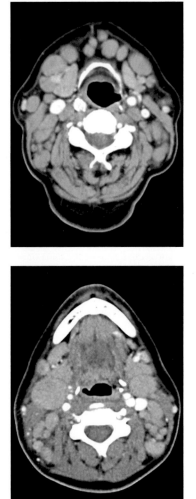

Fig. 10.4 Cervical lymphoma in a woman with CLL. Postcontrast CT. There is a marked increase in the size and number of cervical lymph nodes, particularly in the anterior and lateral cervical triangles. The lymph nodes are iso- or hyperdense to the surrounding muscles.

Fig. 10.5 NHL. Postcontrast CT. There are numerous and markedly enlarged lymph nodes in the submandibular and parajugular spaces, and posterior to the sternocleidomastoid muscle. They are round to oval in shape, show homogeneous enhancement after contrast administration, and are hyperdense to surrounding muscles.

neous enhancement after contrast administration ● Central necrosis in Hodgkin disease shows high T2-weighted signal intensity and very low T1-weighted signal intensity ● Affected nodes show high T2-weighted signal intensity after USPIO administration.

▶ **Pathognomonic findings**
Lymph nodes are increased in size and number ● L/T ratio < 2 ● Frequent bilateral nodal conglomerates ● Lymph nodes in Hodgkin disease usually show homogeneous density and signal intensity ● Some lymph nodes in NHL exhibit central necrosis ● Hodgkin disease and NHL cannot be positively distinguished from each other by their imaging features alone ● NHL is more often generalized, whereas Hodgkin disease tends to be localized.

Clinical Aspects

▶ **Typical presentation**
Multiple, usually bilateral, painless cervical masses ● Night sweats ● Fever ● Weight loss ● Possible cutaneous manifestations ● Pruritus.

▶ **Treatment options**
Treatment depends on stage, cell type, and patient's age ● Radiotherapy alone is usually adequate for low-grade NHL and Hodgkin disease in a favorable prognosis group ● Intermediate prognosis group or high-grade NHL requires chemotherapy and radiation ● Combination chemotherapy is indicated for Hodgkin disease with an unfavorable prognosis ● Recurrent Hodgkin disease requires bone-marrow or stem-cell transplantation.

▶ **Course and prognosis**
Hodgkin disease: Cure rates of 50–90%, depending on the prognostic group ● Increased risk of treatment-induced second neoplasm.
Low-grade NHL: Slow progression ● Usually reaches a generalized stage that is incurable ● Survival time 2–10 years ● 50% cure rate in the localized stage.
High-grade NHL: Rapid progression ● Localized in 10–15% of cases, generalized in 85–90% ● Short survival time without treatment ● Approximately 50% cure rate in treated cases.

▶ **What does the clinician want to know?**
Which lymph node groups are affected? ● Involvement of extranodal organs ● Neurovascular changes.

Differential Diagnosis

Sarcoidosis	– Diffuse cervical lymphadenopathy in some cases
	– Usually associated with mediastinal or hilar lymph node enlargement
	– Coarse calcifications in some lesions
Metastases	– Involvement based on lymphatic drainage of primary tumor
	– Large lymph node metastases often show central necrosis
Cervical lymphadenitis	– Infectious manifestations
	– Painful lymph node swelling
	– Possible central cavitation

Tips and Pitfalls

Physiological structures (e.g., scalene and digastric muscles, submandibular gland) may be mistaken for enlarged lymph nodes ● Differentiation is aided by coronal and sagittal scans or reformatted images ● Lymphoma and lymph node metastases are often indistinguishable by their imaging features alone, without regard for the clinical findings.

Selected References

Fishman EK et al. CT of lymphoma: spectrum of disease. Radiographics 1991; 11 (4): 647–669

Kaji AV et al. Imaging of cervical lymphadenopathy. Semin Ultrasound CT MRI 1997; 18: 220–249

Mende U et al. Sonographische Kriterien für Staging und Verlaufskontrolle bei malignen Lymphomen. Radiologe 1997; 37: 19–26

Definition

▶ **Epidemiology**
Frequency of metastases to various regions: Oropharynx 70%, hypopharynx 70%, nasopharynx 60%, major salivary glands 50%, oral cavity 45%, middle ear 30%, larynx 25%, nose and paranasal sinuses 20% ● Forty percent of metastatically involved lymph nodes are smaller than 1 cm.

▶ **Etiology, pathophysiology, pathogenesis**
Most primary tumors arise in the head and neck region ● Most lymphatic metastases, especially in the Waldeyer ring, are from squamous cell carcinoma ● Lymphoepithelial tumors also metastasize to the head and neck ● Metastases from malignant melanoma are less common ● The route of metastasis depends on the lymphatic drainage of the primary tumor.

Regional lymph node metastases (TNM classification) from head and neck tumors, excluding thyroid tumors:
- N1: Metastasis in a single ipsilateral lymph node ≤ 3 cm.
- N2a: Metastasis in a single ipsilateral lymph node 3–6 cm.
- N2b: Metastasis in multiple ipsilateral lymph nodes ≤ 6 cm.
- N2c: Metastasis in bilateral or contralateral lymph nodes ≤ 6 cm.
- N3: Metastasis in a lymph node > 6 cm.

AJCC classification of lymph nodes by levels:
- Level I: Cranial to the hyoid bone, caudal to the mylohyoid muscle, anterior to the posterior border of the submandibular gland.
- Level II: Extends craniocaudally from the skull base to the hyoid bone, behind the posterior border of the submandibular gland, anterior to the posterior border of the sternocleidomastoid muscle.
- Level III: Extends craniocaudally from the hyoid bone to the inferior border of the cricoid cartilage, anterior to the posterior border of the sternocleidomastoid muscle.
- Level IV: Extends craniocaudally from the inferior border of the cricoid cartilage to the level of the clavicles, anterior to a line between the posterior border of the sternocleidomastoid muscle and the posterolateral border of the scalenus anterior.
- Level V: Extends craniocaudally from the skull base to the clavicles, behind a line between the posterior border of the sternocleidomastoid muscle and the posterolateral border of the scalenus anterior.
- Level VI: Extends craniocaudally from the inferior border of the hyoid bone to the manubrium sterni, medial to the common carotid artery.
- Level VII: Caudal to the superior border of the manubrium sterni, medial to the common carotid artery.

Imaging Signs

▶ **Modality of choice**
Contrast-enhanced CT, MRI with USPIO.

Fig. 10.6 Metastasis. Axial CT of a patient with carcinoma of the tongue shows numerous enlarged lymph nodes in the cervical neurovascular sheath on the right side with indentation of the internal jugular vein and posterior displacement of the sternocleidomastoid muscle. Note the round, enhancing sublingual lymph node.

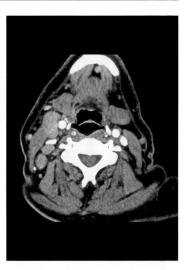

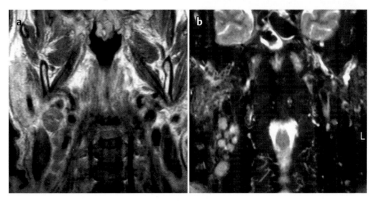

Fig. 10.7 a, b Coronal T1-weighted MR image (**a**) shows multiple enlarged lymph nodes in the right side of the neck. The nodes have intermediate to low signal intensity and are distributed along the neurovascular sheath. STIR sequence (**b**) shows markedly increased signal intensity in the metastatic lymph nodes on the right side.

▶ **CT findings**
Transverse diameter of lymph node > 1 cm ● Round shape ● Enhancement after contrast administration may be homogeneous, inhomogeneous, or peripheral ● Central hypodense cavitation may occur ● Absence of hilar fat sign.

▶ **MRI findings**
Enlarged, rounded lymph nodes ● Three or more lymph nodes in a clustered arrangement ● Nonspecific signal characteristics on plain T1- and T2-weighted images ● Central tumor necrosis is hyperintense on T2-weighted images and markedly hypointense to the peripheral rim on T1-weighted images, especially after gadolinium administration ● MRI with USPIO provides high accuracy and sensitivity ● Eccentric or central lymph node areas with high T2-weighted signal intensity after USPIO represent tumor-affected areas.

▶ **Sonographic findings**
Rounded lymph node shape (L/T ratio < 2) ● Hypoechoic ● Regressive changes ● No hilar echo ● Ill-defined margins in some cases ● Scant vascularity ● Irregular vascularization pattern (spoked wheel) in color duplex images ● Intranodal resistance index higher than in benign lymph nodes (RI > 0.8).

▶ **Pathognomonic findings**
Lymph node > 4 cm ● L/T ratio < 2 ● Clustered lymph node arrangement ● Absence of hilar fat sign ● Central necrosis ● Central, eccentric, or generalized increase of T2-weighted signal intensity after USPIO administration.

Clinical Aspects

▶ **Typical presentation**
Firm, painless, rounded mass ● Superficial lymph node metastases are occult in 10% of cases due to their small size ● Difficult to palpate in deeper regions.

▶ **Treatment options**
Surgical excision of the primary tumor and neck dissection to remove affected lymph node groups.
Radical neck dissection: Resection of the lymph node groups at levels I–V (p. 249) along with the sternocleidomastoid muscle, internal jugular vein, and accessory nerve.
Modified radical neck dissection: Resection of the lymph node groups at levels I–V (p. 249) while sparing the muscle, vein, and nerve.
Selective neck dissection: Selective removal of one or more lymph node groups at levels I–V (p. 249).
Postoperative radiotherapy.

▶ **Course and prognosis**
Undifferentiated carcinomas have a higher incidence of metastasis than well-differentiated carcinomas ● Fixation of lymph nodes implies poor prognosis ● Cases with invasion of the common or internal carotid artery are inoperable ● Lymph node metastases reduce the long-term survival rate by up to 50%.

▶ **What does the clinician want to know?**
Location of enlarged and/or suspicious lymph nodes based on AJCC levels (p. 249) ● Invasion of neurovascular structures ● Organ involvement.

Lymph Nodes

Differential Diagnosis

Cervical lymphoma	– Often difficult to distinguish from lymph node metastasis
	– Affected nodes tend to form conglomerates
	– Central necrosis is common in Hodgkin disease
Jugular vein thrombosis	– Tubular mass in the internal jugular vein
Cervical lymphadenitis	– Infectious manifestations
	– Painful lymph node swelling
	– Possible central cavitation

Tips and Pitfalls

Physiological structures (e.g., scalene and digastric muscles, submandibular gland) may be mistaken for enlarged lymph nodes ● Differentiation is aided by coronal and sagittal scans or reformatted images ● Lymphoma and lymph node metastases are often indistinguishable by their imaging features alone, without regard for the clinical findings.

Selected References

Curtin HD et al. Comparison of CT and MR imaging in staging of neck metastases. Radiology 1998; 207: 123–130

Scheidler JH et al. Radiological evaluation of lymph node metastases in patients with cervical cancer. A meta-analysis. J Amer med Ass 1997; 278: 1096–1101

Sigal R et al. Lymph node metastases from head and neck squamous cell carcinoma: MR imaging with ultrasmall superparamagnetic iron oxide particles (Sinerem MR) – results of a phase-III multicenter clinical trial. Eur Radiol 2002; 12: 1104–1113

Som PM et al. Imaging based nodal classification for evaluation of neck metastatic lymphadenopathy. AJR 2000; 174: 837–844